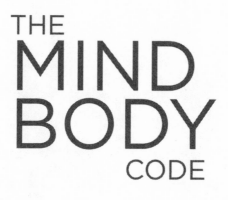

THE
MIND
BODY
CODE

THE
MIND
BODY
CODE

How to Change the Beliefs
that Limit Your Health,
Longevity, and Success

DR. MARIO MARTINEZ

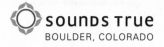
SOUNDS TRUE
BOULDER, COLORADO

Sounds True
Boulder, CO 80306

Published 2014

Book design by Beth Skelley

Printed in the United States of America

Library of Congress Cataloging-in-Publication Data
Martinez, Mario E.
  The mindbody code: how to change the beliefs that limit your health, longevity,
and success / Mario E. Martinez.
    pages cm
  Includes bibliographical references and index.
  ISBN 978-1-62203-199-3
  1. Mind and body. 2. Optimism. I. Title.
  BF151.M37 2014
  158.1—dc23
                        2014020150

Ebook ISBN 978-1-62203-223-5

10 9 8 7 6 5 4 3 2 1

Para mi madre, la mujer que me protegió en mi pasado y facilito mi futuro. Descansa en paz.

Contents

CONTENTS

Foreword

have found a true kindred spirit in Dr. Mario Martinez. His work arrived in my life at just the right time, giving me the scientific basis and language I can use to explain things that I've long known but could never truly articulate in a life-changing way. I am continuously enthralled by the way Dr. Martinez explains how and why our beliefs are stronger than our genes. His explanation of biocognition—how our culture, beliefs, and immune systems all operate in a seamless unity that creates our experience of health and happiness—offers a new language that explains so much about what I've experienced as a physician who has spent decades on the front lines of women's health. I delight in having discovered this language, so when Dr. Martinez asked me to write this foreword, I was deeply honored. Just as *The MindBody Code* will help you identify and change the meaning of the cultural portals in your own life, I want to share with you how his work has informed my view on many topics that are extremely important to me, including women's experiences of childbirth, perceptions around breast cancer and mammography, our standard retirement age, myths of what aging is like, and ageism in general.

As a past president of the American Holistic Medical Association, I have long been aware of the power our minds and beliefs have to either heal or harm. I have seen how people who have near-death experiences and other medical "anomalies," such as spontaneous remission from cancer, are dismissed by the medical community because they have experienced something that mainstream medicine doesn't believe is true. In the words of the late Linus Pauling, PhD, "What we're not up on, we tend to be down on." I have seen how the culture of medicine—supposedly based on science—is as blind to the limitations of its own worldview as a fundamentalist group that believes God has chosen them to interpret reality for everyone else. But I have experienced the uncanny accuracy found in the wisdom of the body, with its astounding ability to get our soul's attention. While writing my book *Mother-Daughter Wisdom,* I nearly went blind in my left eye. In Traditional Chinese Medicine, our eyes are on the liver meridian—which is associated with feelings of anger. I was writing about my childhood, and long-suppressed anger at my own mother was finally arising so I could see it. While it was deemed medically impossible, with loads of vitamin C and a series of adult insights that allowed me to acknowledge and release the anger of the unhealed child within me, I recovered my full vision.

Dr. Martinez's new language of biocognition—how our culture affects our biology—provides a basis for so many insights into health. As an ob/gyn physician, I apply these insights to the cultural rite of passage known as "childbirth." The benefits of natural childbirth in a supportive setting are irrefutable. The presence of a supportive woman—known as a *doula*—during labor has been shown to offer biological benefits that reduce the risk of a Caesarean birth by 50 percent. Care from a doula also shortens labor by several hours. The chief researcher on this topic, Dr. John Kennell, points out that if doulas were present during all labors, it would save the country at least $3 billion a year in unnecessary costs from epidural anesthesia and the complications that often ensue. As he says, "If this were a drug, it would be unethical not to use it." A C-section is major abdominal surgery, and the World Health Organization states that, for this surgery, a rate greater than 15 percent is counterproductive and harmful. And yet, the Caesarean birth rate in most US hospitals—as well as in many other countries—is now 30 to 50 percent. The high rate of unnecessary interventions, such as elective labor inductions, has not only resulted in a significant increase in prematurity, but has also led to an epidemic of surgical births that, in the last twenty years, has doubled the maternal mortality rate.

When I was actively involved in obstetrics, I did everything in my power to support women who desired childbirths free from undue interventions. I put myself in the position of a warrior, protecting the vulnerability of pregnant and laboring women and standing up for their right to birth normally. Despite all my efforts, I found that the culture of fear around birth, and the interventions that stem from it, dominated the valiant efforts of warriors like me. We champion birthing for its amazing potential to be the most potent rite of passage into wisdom and power available to a woman—a potency Dr. Martinez would call the "healing field."

Here's the thing that *The MindBody Code* pointed out to me so powerfully: Doctors aren't to blame. Women aren't to blame. Everyone is simply operating under the unconscious spells of their cultural programming. The inherited cultural belief that birthing is a disaster waiting to happen—which is aided and abetted by the media—is a very potent cultural portal for pregnant women. It is passed down seamlessly from the previous generation—unless, of course, you happen to belong to a subculture of individuals who have experienced birthing with pleasure and power. Then there is hope for waking from the spell of cultural conditioning.

Here's another potent cultural portal: breast cancer screening. Unbeknownst to most women, Breast Cancer Awareness Month (October) was initiated by a mammogram company thirty years ago. Thus was born one of the most successful campaigns for breast cancer screening ever—all based on the notion that early detection saves lives. This is a powerful cultural belief that has been shown to have fundamental flaws. The results from a landmark study by A. Blyer, MD, and H. Gilbert Welch, MD, were published in 2012 in a *New England Journal of Medicine* article entitled "Effect of Three Decades of Screening Mammography on Breast Cancer Incidence." The researchers estimate that, in the last thirty years, breast cancer was overdiagnosed in 1.3 million women, as screening detected tumors that would have gone away on their own or never become clinically significant. In 2008 alone, seventy thousand women were overdiagnosed with so-called breast cancers that were actually *ductal carcinoma in situ (DCIS)*—which is *not* cancer and which doesn't progress. Yes, some women are helped by mammogram screening: about eight cases per hundred thousand. Compare that to the 114 per hundred thousand who were overdiagnosed.

Before this new data was available, the US Preventive Services Task Force recommended that women younger than fifty decrease the frequency of mammography, noting that the potential harms of overdiagnosis—such as undergoing chemotherapy, surgery, and radiation treatments—outweighed the benefits. Despite the fact that this recommendation was based on an unbiased review of decades of accumulated data, a huge public outcry ensued. There is a profound cultural belief that breasts are two pre-malignant lesions sitting on our chests and that our only hope of survival is regular screening. Because of this, the recommendation was criticized as an assault on women's health and a poll published in *USA Today* found that despite these new guidelines, 84 percent of women who were thirty-five to forty-nine years old planned to ignore them!

Dr. Martinez would call this the triumph of cultural beliefs over everything else—even science. I notice that whenever I write about the risks of mammography on my Facebook page, it really doesn't matter what the facts are. There are always a few women who view this kind of information as "dangerous." It is as though, by pointing out the whole truth that we have the power to be healthy or sick, I am actually risking someone's life.

Dr. Lisa Rosenbaum wrote about her experience working in a women's cardiology clinic where every new patient was asked, "What is the number one killer of women?"

Ms. S., a middle-aged woman with high blood pressure and hyperlipidemia [high cholesterol] answered in a way that sticks with me. "I know that the right answer is heart disease" she said, eyeing me as if facing an irresistible temptation, "but I'm still going to say breast cancer." . . . Ms. S.'s response short-circuited my statistical litany [that heart diseases take more women's lives than all types of cancer combined and is largely preventable]. Her sense of risk was clearly less about fact than about feeling. Would more facts really address those feelings? (NEJM, February 13, 2014, p. 595)

The answer to Dr. Rosenbaum's question is, of course, a resounding "No." When it comes to our health, our cultural beliefs are far more potent than any other factor. They are nearly impervious to any fact of any kind. But that doesn't mean cultural beliefs can't be changed.

One of the big ones for baby boomers right now is the "retirement age" of sixty-five. This appears to be some kind of culturally approved time when you are supposed to retire to a golf community in Florida and step out of useful life. It happens just when you truly feel a sense of mastery with whatever skills you have so far cultivated in your life. Why this retirement-at-sixty-five portal? Where did that come from? My own research revealed that this retirement age was instituted in Germany by Kaiser Otto Von Bismarck as a way to give people a state-funded pension so they could rest before they died. This was in 1880. At the time, the average life expectancy after you turned sixty-five was only eighteen months. It's now twenty-four years! Clearly this is a cultural portal that requires some significant updating.

I was introduced to *The MindBody Code* when I was in the middle of writing about women and how to remain "ageless" for a book called *Goddesses Never Age: The Secret Prescription for Vitality, Radiance, and Joy.* Dr. Martinez's ideas were the missing link I had been looking for. Getting older needn't be associated with physical deterioration. His phrase, "Growing older is inevitable, aging is optional" became a mantra that I now use all the time. My mother hiked the Appalachian trail in her seventies. Then at the age of eighty-four, she hiked to the Mount Everest base camp, which requires walking a great distance uphill—with access to half of the oxygen present at sea level. I knew that her physical prowess was not "genetic" because her mother died of a heart attack at the age of sixty-eight. Her father died at age seventy-five from heart disease. From watching my mother, I know that it is her joy of movement and the outdoors and hiking that is the key to her health and wellbeing. Like the centenarians studied so thoroughly by Dr. Martinez—whose stories you will find in this book—my mother doesn't go to doctors. Nor does she hang around with sick, old people whose conversations revolve around doctor visits or aches and pains. In fact, she had to pay a large fine for not buying a prescription drug plan when she technically became a "senior citizen." Her reasoning was simple: she wasn't on any prescription drugs so she didn't purchase a plan. It was a turning point for me to learn from Dr. Martinez's studies of healthy centenarians. What a revelation to have him articulate something that I've always known, that gerontology is the study of the pathology of aging—not the study of healthy aging.

Dr. Martinez's work also gives me permission to refuse to do something that I intuitively knew I needed to stop doing: Giving out my age—ever. Because in this culture, we use age as a cage. And that "cage" starts early; my hairdresser turned twenty-nine this year and her friends are feeding her fears of a dreaded thirtieth birthday. I am stronger and healthier now than I was in my twenties. When I work out on the elliptical trainer, I always enter my age as forty because I don't want some algorithm based on the pathology of aging to tell me how I'm supposed to feel. Now, when asked for my age, I say the following, "My biological age is thirty-five and my wisdom age is at least 300." Talk about freeing! And I have told my children that I will never celebrate a "milestone" birthday again. Others, like Gloria Steinem, can continue that tradition if they wish. Not me.

I have said a lot about how *The MindBody Code* has impacted my own work and life because I know that it can also profoundly impact yours. You don't need to stay caged in a life of culturally approved "known misery" that keeps you from experiencing a lifetime of wonder, health, and joy. You have within you the power to reinvent yourself at any age or stage—no matter what your circumstances.

Dr. Martinez has spent a lifetime figuring out precisely how to change the beliefs and cultural imprints that keep us stuck. With his work, we can get on with what he calls the "exalted emotions" of joy and love and happiness—procured through means that free us from paying a price for them with our bodies, relationships, and health. *The MindBody Code* extends a thrilling invitation to step into a life more fulfilling than you ever dreamed possible. The roadmap is right here in these pages.

Thank you, Dr. Martinez. Thank you.

—Christiane Northrup, MD

Women's health visionary and author of the *New York Times* bestsellers
The Wisdom of Menopause and *Women's Bodies, Women's Wisdom*

November, 2014

Introduction

Have you ever read a motivational or self-help book that promised you a life of abundance in ten easy steps? Maybe one that whispered a "secret" based on positive thinking and intentions? Have you attended workshops that you thought had the potential to transform your life, to help you overcome some of the challenges you wrestle with and can never seem to resolve? After your initial rush of hope and excitement when you turned the first pages of the book or entered the workshop space, what happened?

If your experience is like that of many, many others, while you may have gleaned some useful ideas, in the end, you did not find your life substantially improved. The persistent, challenging behavior patterns and unwanted thinking that led you to seek solutions to begin with are still in place. Despite the best intentions of the authors you read and the workshop leaders you met—and your own earnest efforts—you still feel stuck. Why is this? Why have your efforts not yielded fruit?

As a clinical neuropsychologist, I spent years searching for answers to these questions and for methods that can effect deep and lasting change. In addition to exploring this in my practice, I traveled the world, studying the ways in which cultural beliefs affect health, happiness, and longevity. Ultimately, I discovered the answer to why popular methods of self-transformation so often fail. It is because good intentions are not sufficient to enable you to access and work with the *mindbody code,* the set of "operating instructions" you embodied while you were growing up and that you reinforce as you move through your life as an adult. To effect real and enduring change, the process of change must itself engage the fullness of the mindbody code.

The mindbody code is the language you learn from your culture that enables you to interpret your world, shape your self-concept, and find meaning in what you do. As you learn to access and shift the code that your mindbody uses to make sense of your world, you will find that it is entirely possible to change unhelpful patterns you may have come to think you will never break free of.

Think about the limitations of a conceptual approach to change. If dysfunctional lifestyles and toxic behaviors could be modified with logical arguments, smokers would quit smoking the moment they learned their habit would most likely kill them. The depressed could be persuaded to lift their mood by noting that there are others with worse problems. All self-sabotaging strategies would cease the instant they were intellectually identified as such. But we know from our own experiences how perplexed we feel when we continue behaving in ways or remaining in relationships that are not in our best interest.

The solution to all your impasses and suffering is not to kill your ego or detach from your negative emotions. You need your ego to deal with the practical aspects of life, and *all* emotions are essential biological information that tells you how your body is responding to the interpretations you make about your circumstances. True sustainable change requires gaining access to the cultural beliefs that deny you the rewards of your courageous commitment to change. It requires a new vision of how your body responds to your beliefs and how you can change those beliefs through an embodied approach.

I have seen this method work in practice again and again, both for my patients and in my own life. I believe that what has emerged from my quest for answers is truly revolutionary, and through witnessing it myself, I can attest that the effectiveness of these methods is not in doubt. Yet this is a journey that requires dedication; I do not claim a quick fix. I wrote this book for those who are willing to look beyond the quick-fix mentality and make a commitment to patience and perseverance. These are the qualities you will need to call upon in order to access the mindbody code that shapes your self-concept and the perceptions you use to interpret your world.

Because the mindbody code breaks significant new ground, understanding and working with it requires learning a new vocabulary, and I will be introducing new terms throughout the book, in italics upon first use. As is the case when you learn any new language, you will encounter words and concepts that are not yet part of your mode of thinking. The word *mindbody* itself, for example, is an expression of the inseparable oneness of mind and body functioning—a fundamental concept in this book.

At first, exposure to these new terms and concepts may trigger some uncertainty and, perhaps, a sense of bewilderment. If this happens to you, it is actually good news! Such feelings of unease are simply emotional feedback telling you that you have reached your *belief horizon,* the edge of your operational consciousness. At that point, you have a choice. You can give in to the unease and return to the *known misery* you have become accustomed to, or you can move forward with the understanding that your *felt puzzlement* is how your brain prepares to incorporate new learning. In other words, the edges of what you presently know need to be shaken up so that new information can enter your knowledge base and expand your vision. This is a good thing.

Working with the mindbody code involves the theory and practice of the new field of *biocognition.* In developing this theory, I have brought together several disciplines from the life sciences that, unfortunately, have not been communicating with one another about the potential benefits of their discoveries. As a result of this disconnection, their findings in the areas of health, well-being, and longevity tend to reach the public in the form of disjointed messages that offer limited practical applications. Psychoneuroimmunology (PNI) investigates how thoughts and emotions affect the immune, nervous, and endocrine systems; medical anthropology observes how cultures shape the concepts of wellness and illness; and Eastern philosophies and Western *contemplative psychology* explore the deeper dimensions of the mind. All of these disciplines are indispensable in studying the complexities of human experience, yet they must be joined together if they are to offer their highest potential. With biocognition, I propose a model of *mind-body-culture* that explores each of these three components within the holism of a single and inseparable entity. I offer an example that will help you start thinking along these lines. When I used to surf, I studied the characteristics of each wave, never forgetting that the waves were inseparable *coauthors*—a term you will become very familiar with as you journey through this book—with their ocean. I invite you to become a wave in a cultural ocean that will offer all the answers if you explore the right questions with an open mind.

Let me reiterate that a change of mindset requires more than intellectually discarding unwanted behavior. It involves accessing the mindbody code that maintains all the dysfunctional patterns related to the behavior. If you attempt to give up smoking without *recontextualizing* (revisioning) the mindbody code distraction that this unwanted behavior provides for you, you will most likely find other distractions (such as overeating or gambling) to fill the vacuum that remains. But as you gradually assimilate the biocognitive strategies I offer here, you will discover the functions of such self-sabotaging distractions and learn how to shift your mindbody understanding to implement permanent change.

The concepts and exercises you will learn in this book are based on how the brain assimilates new ways of thinking and interpreting, rather than on what may feel comfortable or easy to understand. This is because the *mindbody code is not based on reason*. Instead, the code interprets the symbols we create based on the subtle cultural beliefs we have been taught. Let me offer an example. A son who loves his abusive father does not reason that he should remove himself from his situation to be free from physical danger. Instead, for that unfortunate child, the abuse he suffers has become a *biosymbol* of love that keeps him tied to the relationship. This dysfunctional mindbody interpretation of love predisposes him to later seek relationships that "speak" abuse fluently. This is not masochism; it is a helpless attempt to seek the only kind of love his mindbody knows. These are the kinds of paradigm-shifting discoveries you will make as you work through the book.

This book is about how to access the mindbody code so that you can change any beliefs you hold that do not serve you well. Your learning journey will require you to relinquish the beliefs that support your suffering and gradually replace them with a consciousness that promotes what I call the *worthy self*. This is an exciting but, at times, demanding pursuit. If you can trust that you know more than you can presently explain, and that you are ready to welcome your birthright to an abundance of love, health, and wealth, you will at last achieve significant positive change.

For the experiential journey on which you are about to embark, I ask you to adopt the outlook of an explorer eagerly moving toward a new vision that will enhance your health and the quality of both your private and social life. Like any explorer, you will encounter obstacles as you work through the book. They will often take the form of the cultural coauthors of your life who share the beliefs you hold that may not be in your best interest. The path will be easiest if you commit to changing your own perceptions of your world rather than convincing others to make such changes. If the coauthors of your world are going to change, it will most likely happen when they have to respond differently to your new behavior.

HOW THIS BOOK IS ORGANIZED

The consciousness-shifting tools I present in this book are divided into thirteen chapters with strategic themes. Although you may approach them based on your immediate needs, I recommend that you read them sequentially, as all the themes are essential and interconnected. You can then decide when it is appropriate to return to a particular chapter and apply its lessons to your surfacing or immediate needs. To get the most from the concepts and techniques you will encounter, I recommend you approach each chapter as if you were practicing a brand new method of learning—and you are. Remain open to applying the lessons in unique ways. This will be a process of breaking some of the old templates you have been living by and embracing the uncertainty of change.

Chapter 1, which shares the title of the book, offers further information on biocognitive theory. At the end of the chapter, you will embark on your first experiential journey, entering the five portals of wellness: safety, love, expression, peace, and spirit.

In chapter 2, you will learn a fundamental principle of biocognitive work. We all experience certain defined *archetypal wounds,* and each one has an associated *healing field* that can be engaged to resolve the wound. You will experience this directly at the end of the chapter.

Chapter 3 departs from the pattern in that it does not contain a practice. This chapter encapsulates the science behind biocognitive theory; I hope you will share my fascination with the emerging research. From there you will move into a discussion of deeply loving relationships in chapter 4, "Guardians of the Heart," and you will become acquainted with such concepts as *vertical* and *horizontal love,* and *belongingness* versus *ownership.*

In chapter 5, I share what I have learned about health and happiness in my study of centenarians, who, no matter their particular culture, have intuitively established identical beliefs that foster their longevity. You will learn what these beliefs are and have a chance to practice working with them.

Chapter 6 introduces the concept of *abundance phobia,* and the lack of self-worth at its root, and includes exercises for building worthiness.

In chapter 7, I share what I learned about wounding when I studied stigmatics for National Geographic. Here you will explore the role of suffering.

Chapter 8, "Forgiveness as Liberation from Self-Entrapment," contains a mindbody process that releases the blocks to forgiveness; and chapter 9, "Psychospiritual Conflicts and Their Resolution," delves into the mindbody code of spiritual beliefs.

Chapter 10, "From Wishful Thinking to Sustainable Action," concerns the ways in which we distract ourselves from our worthiness, and contains practices to change self-distractive behavior. In chapter 11, you will learn to recognize *portals of synchronicity,* opportunities to engage what I call the *drift.* Here you will find tools with which to explore out-of-order events.

Chapter 12 concerns the vitally important topic of creating your own subcultures of wellness—people to surround yourself with who will support you in your transformative efforts. Finally, chapter 13 offers an array of navigational tools, inner guides you can draw upon to keep you always on the path toward greater health, happiness, and love.

❖ ❖ ❖

If you are willing to explore empowerment when you are afraid, creativity when you are deprived, and self-validation when you are in doubt, you are ready to learn the mindbody code.

Let's begin!

The Mindbody Code

iocognition confirms what you may have already intuitively suspected is a universal truth: your cultural beliefs can make you ill and rob you of your joy. You may simply have lacked the scientific evidence or social support you needed in order to know this for sure. If you have been emotionally wounded by your travels through life, beleaguered by the thieves of love, the biocognitive lessons in this book are your portal to a new journey, one that will empower you to realize your personal greatness.

That the mind affects the body has been well established. The new science of biocognition also recognizes the *cultural* components that affect the mind. Based on the latest scientific studies of healthy brains, healthy longevity, and a strong sense of self-worth, biocognition debunks some very persistent myths: that we are victims of our genetics; that *aging* is an inevitable process of deterioration; and that the life sciences can simply choose to ignore the influence of culture on human health and well-being.

The lessons I will share with you throughout this book did not come easily to me. As a clinical neuropsychologist, I was trained in several very unhelpful practices. I was taught to identify pathology; to confirm a model that interprets life as a constant struggle to maintain health and battle illness; and to view with disdain any theory about mind and body that cannot be measured with established tools. I was trained in a world where gerontologists study the pathology of aging rather than the *wellness* of growing older, and where the pharmaceutical industry entices health care providers to believe the delusion that we are mere biochemical beings and the hapless victims of our genes.

With the language of biocognition, I describe a very different world.

BRINGING UNITY TO DIVERGENT SYSTEMS

With few exceptions, the interdisciplinary field of psychoneuroimmunology (PNI) investigates how thoughts and emotions affect the nervous, immune, and endocrine systems—as if we existed in a laboratory void of cultural context. Medical anthropology principally looks at how cultures conceptualize illness, as if we functioned in a biological void. And most theologies preach divinity with little concern for the transient body that houses our eternal spirit. These disjointed approaches to understanding who we are and what we do with life are necessary, but none is sufficient to embrace the totality that makes us greater than our parts.

Biocognitive theory proposes a paradigm in which consciousness develops in a cultural context that has greater impact on our wellness than do our genes. The good news from the science of wellness, as well as from contemplative studies, is that we can learn much from the *outliers* who defy conventional parameters of mind, body, and spirit. Outliers are those people who deviate from the norms of human behavior established through mechanistic rules. The emerging fields of integrative medicine, embodied anthropology, *cultural neuroscience,* and contemplative psychology are providing persuasive evidence of our power to heal and embrace joy—*sustainable* joy—while confirming that reaching our greatest potential is not "too good to be true."

On our pioneering biocognitive journey toward wellness, we will not fall victim to the usual New Age promises of finding happiness simply by sending good intentions to the universe. Instead, I propose that we achieve what we wish at a speed determined by our cultural beliefs and by the strength of the actions we take that confirm our intrinsic worthiness. In fact, we should deemphasize our quest for a happiness that is dependent on external circumstances, and instead redirect our commitments to an *internal joy* that cannot be plucked from our grasp by the vicissitudes of life.

PARADIGM SHIFT

As we enter this exciting, uncharted territory together, let's examine what usually happens when we are confronted with new information that could challenge our beliefs. In his book *The Structure of Scientific Revolutions,* Thomas Kuhn tells us that science does not progress by simply adding new data to its existing theories. Instead, when new evidence challenges an existing theory, science discards what can no longer be supported and reconstructs the theory to be consistent with the new evidence. Kuhn coined the term *paradigm shift* to illustrate the robust change that takes place under these circumstances. But he also cautioned that such shifts do not happen without resistance. As the mindbody code entails a paradigm shift, it is worth taking a moment to explore this.

When a new theory is formed to accommodate information that contradicts an old theory, first there is disdain—the new theory and its proponents are met with scorn. This is followed by doubt about the new theory's validity. Finally, when the old theory can no longer be defended, the paradigm shifts into acceptance of the new evidence.

For example, when Galileo, who is considered the father of modern science, was able to confirm Copernicus's assertion that the earth was not the center of the universe, as people believed in the seventeenth century, he was put under house arrest by order of the Inquisition and forced to recant his position. Only when his work was published after his death was the disdain for his theory replaced by doubt. And that doubt finally progressed to the paradigm shift in which the sun rather than the earth was accepted as the center of the universe—a heliocentric versus geocentric paradigm. Of course, we now further accept that the sun is only the center of our solar system, not of the entire universe, a further paradigm shift necessitated by scientific discoveries over the intervening centuries.

This slow process of mindset shifts illustrates that our beliefs and behavioral patterns are not relinquished easily. This applies even when we know intellectually that our beliefs and behaviors are less than healthy. This reluctance to change what we consider "known" results from the investments we have made—emotionally, intellectually, and financially—is our personal paradigm.

When we apply this to biocognition, paradoxically enough, we tend to experience more anxiety with *anticipated joy* than with *known misery*. But as we gain fluency in the biocognitive mindbody code, we can move past anxiety and resistance. We can shift our paradigm from living as disdaining disciples of known pain and doubting skeptics of anticipated joy to becoming accepting masters of abundance.

Now let's move from poetics to practicality. I want you to learn to *live* a language that produces results. And you can—if you are willing to replace your fear with the love of discovery. I mention this caveat because my years of clinical practice have taught me that it is easier to heal an illness or change a dysfunctional behavior than it is to confront the people or conditions that support our known misery. For example, I have seen an alarming number of patients who choose to surrender to their illnesses, and in some cases die, rather than assert their emotional boundaries. It is also fascinating to note that such self-sabotaging processes are not conscious, and that these patients will vigorously deny they are sabotaging themselves even when they are confronted with compelling evidence. I am not implying here that illness is a simple matter of being unassertive; there are many variables that contribute to disease. But healing cannot occur if we do not accept our own worthiness—that we are worth healing, even if doing so might shake up our view of the world and how we interact with others. A cure may require external interventions such as psychotherapy, medication, or surgery, but healing requires an internal paradigm shift from fear to love.

Biocognition is more than a theory or a practice. It is a way of life, and this is because each of us is more than a sentient body and a thinking mind. We are individual *living fields of information* that can make sense of who we are by means of the symbols we create from our experiences. Thus, our experiences are embodied interpretations called *biosymbols*, communicated in a *bioinformational field* shared by the communicators—the individual fields converge into a shared field. These two concepts form the terrain of what I call *portals of wellness*.

A *biosymbol* is a word, image, memory, or belief that has been given a cultural interpretation that affects our biology. For example, the word "stupid" is a symbol. It becomes a *bio*symbol, which we experience as physical sensations and emotions, when someone uses the word to describe our own actions.

THE FIVE PORTALS OF WELLNESS

We experience our cultural history through the biosymbols we create, and we communicate biosymbols with both implicit and explicit language. We say things like "I can't stomach that," "My heart's not in it," "I want peace of mind," and many other expressions representing the *mindbody biosymbols* we use to convey our inner and outer world. I propose five areas of the mindbody space that manifest our most essential biosymbols. These range from our need for safety to our quest for spirituality. I call these areas *portals* because they are gates of expression of the *total being:* causes that cannot be attributed to specific physical locations.

It is essential to note that the correlations I make in this model between areas of the body and specific illnesses are not to be interpreted as linear cause and effect. They are not. Here we are in the realm of mindbody expressions of disharmonies.

The First Portal: Safety

The first portal covers a biosymbolic area from the feet to the belly. The physiological expression of this portal is most evident when there is a threat to our physical or emotional safety; a fight-or-flight response is triggered to stop digestion and send extra blood to the legs. In times of perceived danger, the mindbody code determines that fighting or running away is more important than digesting food.

The positive side of this portal is the sense of comfort, delight, and calmness we feel at the end of a lovely meal with close friends. And so we get our first glimpse of biosymbols as coauthored mindbody interpretations responding to internal and external conditions.

The Second Portal: Love

The second portal extends from the solar plexus to the upper chest, and it expresses the biosymbols of love. There is a strong correlation between heart conditions and emotional losses. The biosymbol of a broken heart can be more than a poetic sentiment; the loss of a partner can increase the onset of cardiac abnormalities.

Conversely, experiments show that love and other positive emotions increase coherence in the rhythmic patterns of the heart rate, one of the indicators of cardiac health.

The Third Portal: Expression

The third portal reflects the biosymbols of expression and emotional freedom. It extends from the neck to the eyebrows, as well as to the arms and hands. Our facial and hand expressions (clearing the throat when lying or when having to convey unpleasant news) and the tones of voice we use (such as when discussing socially disturbing content or confronting a feared authority) are all examples of how the third portal manifests biosymbols related to expression.

Although there is no decisive, empirical evidence of this, some clinicians suspect there may be a connection between difficulties in vocalizing feelings and thyroid problems. It has been suggested that, in addition to genetic factors, women may suffer from thyroid disorders more than men because of cultural conditions that discourage them from expressing themselves freely.

The Fourth Portal: Peace

The fourth portal encompasses the area from the forehead to the crown of the head. We experience our thoughts as if they were coming from inside our heads. And although cognition is a collaborative function of mind and body, the forehead seems to be the biosymbolic portal of our mental processes. Expressions such as "I am thinking so much that my head hurts" and "My mind is at peace," as well as tension headaches resulting from excessive worrying, are but a few examples of fourth portal manifestations.

The Fifth Portal: Spirit

This spiritual portal is the most difficult to describe using linear language because of its nonlocal essence. In other words, it does not have a set location, and it does not travel through time and space. Yet we can still give the spiritual portal a metaphorical presence to unify the mental activities emanating from our physical body with a metaphysical entity that transcends our mortality. Poetics such as "spiritual death," "poor of spirit," and "the eternal spirit" are some attempts to express what we intuit but cannot describe.

❖ ❖ ❖

Interestingly, the biosymbolic portals seem to be interwoven in a hierarchical and synergistic architecture: safety forms the foundation upon which love can express itself with peace, and transcend in spirit.

PREPARING FOR THE EXPERIENTIAL TOOLS

Following your brief introduction to a new paradigm that includes biosymbolic language and portals of wellness, it is time for you to begin working with these concepts yourself. The mindbody code is eminently practical, and I devote much of this book to teaching you how to work with it to create the life changes you desire. At the end of each chapter, I have created opportunities for you to begin to assimilate the concepts of biocognition. As you gain fluency with the terminology, you will progress from understanding the theory to experiencing the practice. There are two fundamental principles to guide you through this transformational journey: the *embodied mind* and the *lived theory.*

The Embodied Mind

To *embody* is to identify how and where cognition is experienced in the body. What physical and emotional sensations do our thoughts trigger, and where does the body manifest the experience? If someone says "I love you" or "I hate you," those symbols (words) become biosymbols when we interpret them through the filter of our cultural beliefs and express them as embodied sensations and emotions. And the following point is key to working with the mindbody code: If we try to modify a belief without attending to the embodiment process, the change will likely be partial and unsustainable. In other words, changing a belief requires a *mindbody recoding process that impacts the cultural meaning that sustains the belief.* To intellectualize change without embodiment is like trying to rate the quality of a wine without tasting it.

The Lived Theory

Living a theory entails embodying its principles in the form of actions. And to sustain a change to live the theory, actions must become rituals.

A ritual is different from a routine. *Routine* is action we take to maintain a level of functioning, whereas *ritual* is meaningful action that defines who we are in our culture. Taking a shower, going to work, shaving, and shopping are examples of routines. Breaking bread with family, celebrations with friends, religious ceremonies, pilgrimages to sacred places, and meditating are examples of rituals. Sadly, a status-driven lifestyle can cause us to confuse egocentric routines with healthy rituals.

In chapter 3, I will explain how cultural beliefs affect the immune system, and in chapter 5, you will learn why healthy rituals, rather than routines, can be stress buffers that counteract the negative effects of social pressures and turbulent times.

The Experiential Language

As is the case when you learn any new language, the concepts and terminology you encounter in each chapter of this book will gain experiential meaning for you through dedicated practice. Biocognitive concepts challenge our *belief horizons* (the limits or edges of our knowing) with experiential tools that can transform dysfunctional patterns into *wellness consciousness.* But the mindbody code is experienced rather than spoken, and it is accessed *incidentally*—through roundabout means—rather than directly. Buddhist teachers present their lessons with similar principles of *incidental learning* through an experiential language.

Say that a master wants to teach his student to experience the meaning of humility. "Wash my feet!" he orders the student.

Feeling insulted, the student responds, "Do you think I am your servant?"

The master retorts, "Well, then, let *me* wash *your* feet."

Here humility is taught indirectly, and its meaning is experienced as a shift of consciousness.

According to biocognitive theory, a belief is a set of learned propensities (predisposed mindbody cultural interpretations) to give context to a perception. Put another way, a belief is a set of cultural assumptions to create meaning. For example, if your culture believes that tall people are intelligent, you will develop a learned propensity to find intelligence in tall people, so you can confirm your assumption. And your belief horizons determine how far the assumptions that maintain that belief can go without being challenged. In this case, you might reach your belief horizon if you learn that an author you consider one of the most brilliant people on earth stands only four feet ten.

Before we can alter a belief that does not serve us well, we must question it at its horizon to defy our old predispositions. This questioning takes place in a contemplative state of calmness, and the conditions that maintain the belief are altered experientially by incidentally accessing the mindbody code. Using a video game to indirectly teach a child eye-motor coordination is an example of *incidental learning*. But I want to clarify that beliefs are not maintained by rigid algorithms. We are not computers that process data; we are sentient fields of bioinformation that seek the greatest contextual relevance possible to find meaning in our world.

To illustrate, a clown preaching in a church would shake up the contextual relevance—a clown's expected context is the circus or a child's birthday party, not a church. But if the clown says to his congregation, "I am your new preacher, and I dressed like a clown to get your attention before I give you my first sermon," he restores contextual relevance.

Greater contextual relevance in that setting would be to have the preacher dress as expected when giving a sermon.

THE FOUNDATION OF PRACTICE: CONTEMPLATIVE OBSERVATION

We will use a contemplative method (observation, not interpretation) to explore how the dysfunctional mindbody scripts we learned from authority figures (what I term our *cultural editors*) manifest throughout the five mindbody portals I introduced in this chapter.

The transition from an alert-interpretation state of awareness (characterized by beta brain waves) to a contemplative-observation consciousness (involving theta brain waves) facilitates the receptiveness and assimilation we need to redefine the implicit beliefs that drive our dysfunctional behavioral patterns. Reading this paragraph, for example, requires an alert state of beta waves. If you were in a deep state of meditation, you would be in a calm state of theta waves. A five-year-old's brain operates predominantly at theta frequencies, which facilitates learning and assimilation of new information, while a teenager's brain functions predominantly at beta frequencies and, as a result, is well suited to questioning new information.

The Contemplative Method

It is now time for you to learn the contemplative method that is the foundation of this life-changing work. This section features my own method, but if you know another technique that allows you to experience deep relaxation, it is fine to use that one instead. If you have never tried a relaxation exercise, be patient if you find that it takes you a bit longer than you expect. The key to reaching a contemplative state of serenity is to *not try* to relax! If you try to relax, most likely it will have the opposite effect because to "try" is to concentrate on a goal rather than to witness a process. Trust that you already experienced deep levels of calm when you were an infant, and forgot how to reenter that state only when you learned how to worry. The contemplative method I teach in this chapter will remind you of what you already know, and is the first step in most of the practices presented in this book.

The object of this contemplative method is threefold. It will enable you to:

❖ witness for yourself the portals of safety, love, expression, peace, and spirit
❖ learn to access the mindbody code
❖ identify patterns of stress and their biosymbols

◇◇◇

The Method—Witnessing and Breathing

Before you begin, here is an important reminder: the mindbody code pathways are accessed indirectly and communicated *experientially*. They do not operate in a linear or intellectual way. Simply reasoning out or wishing for a solution will not change the conditions that maintain dysfunctional patterns. This is a key reason why self-destructive behavior does not change as a result of fear tactics or appeals to logic.

Please read the following instructions several times until you can do the technique with your eyes closed. Do not worry about following the steps perfectly. Trust that with practice, you will develop the proficiency you need.

Please note that this experiential exercise will introduce you to all five of the wellness portals, but you do not have to explore them all at once. You can practice working with one portal at a time for as long as you wish, or you can practice with all five portals during one sitting. The method works best when you adjust it to your personal preference and needs.

❖ Sit in a quiet place, in a comfortable chair or on the floor. If you choose to sit on the floor, elevate yourself on the edge of a pillow to take any pressure off your back. Always sit with your back against a wall. (Sensing that your back is protected is the mindbody code for embodied safety.) If you choose a chair, use one with a solid back.

❖ Close your eyes. Keep your back straight without straining. Tilt your head slightly forward. Relax your jaw and drop your shoulders.

❖ Feel your back touching the back of the chair, or sense your back resting against the solid wall.

❖ Feel your body being held by the chair or the floor. Release the belly and pelvic muscles that tighten when you're standing. Trust that the solidness holding you in place will sustain you. (Sensing solidness holding your body is the mindbody code for *embodied support.*)

❖ Allow yourself to feel gratitude for the consciousness of safety and support you have created. Let this emerging gratitude slowly permeate your body. (Gratitude is an *exalted emotion*—a term we will explore more fully later in the book—that promotes receptiveness. The manifested experience of gratitude is the mindbody code for *embodied acceptance* and *assimilation of wellness.*)

❖ Witness your breathing as if you were watching a film. Do not interfere with the rhythm; simply be aware of your breathing pattern.

◇◇◇◇◇◇◇◇◇◇◇◇◇◇◇◇◇◇◇◇◇◇◇◇◇◇◇◇◇◇◇

Explore the Five Portals
THE FIRST PORTAL: BELLY TO FEET

❖ Repeat in your mind the word *safety* while focusing attention on your belly and your legs. Every few breaths, repeat the word *safety* like a mantra, and begin to witness your belly and legs as a unified field.

❖ Do not expect anything or try to modify any reaction you may have. Your only task is to make the mindbody connection between the word *safety* and the first portal.

❖ If memories or emotions surface, witness them without attachment and let them pass. If tension builds in the safety portal, simply witness the sensation and breathe as if you were sending a gentle wave of fresh oxygen to the tense area.

❖ Let your breathing embrace the area rather than trying to relax the muscles in the area. (This breathing-to-an-area technique is the mindbody code for *embodied release*.) Although you can't literally breathe directly into an area beyond the lungs, breathing as if you can indirectly triggers the relaxation response to the tense area.

❖ After a few minutes of doing these steps, change the mantra from *safety* to "I am safety," and follow the same witnessing procedure for another few minutes.

❖ Now engage the final mantra, "I take safety wherever I go," for the same amount of time and with the same steps as for the other two mantras.

❖ After completing the three mantras, you can choose to end the exercise by counting from one to ten, opening your eyes, and slowly reorienting yourself before getting up. Or you can move on to the next portal.

THE NEXT THREE PORTALS

❖ The next three portals, love, expression, and peace, are experienced using the same procedure as for the safety portal.

❖ Each time, move from the mantra expressing the specific portal (repeating its name every few breaths) to the mantra "I am [the portal]," and finally to the mantra "I take [the portal] wherever I go."

❖ Proceed from the love mantra (the solar plexus and upper chest), to the mantra "I am love," and finally to "I take love wherever I go."

❖ Begin with the expression mantra (arms, hands, and neck to eyebrows), move to "I am expression" mantra, and then repeat "I take expression wherever I go."

❖ Go from the peace mantra (forehead to crown), to "I am peace," to "I take peace wherever I go."

❖ After you complete the exercise for the fourth mantra, if you choose to, you can move on to the fifth and final portal.

THE FIFTH PORTAL: SPIRIT

The procedure for this portal is different from the others because, as I mentioned before, the spiritual dimension does not have locality and does not reside in time and space; it has a nonlocal presence in an infinite realm. Thoughts, sensations, and feelings are amorphous glimpses of consciousness that take form and identity when we attempt to describe them. Spirit, however, is beyond consciousness and cannot be accessed directly. We can only experience the *undulations of spirit*—the reflection of its presence. (I will explain the concept of undulations in the next section, Going Deeper.)

❖ Before starting the spirit mantra, scan your body and witness what is going on without attempting to intervene or change anything. Just be aware of the process. Whatever thoughts, sensations, or feelings surface, notice them and allow them to move on.

❖ Focus on your breathing and begin to repeat the spirit mantra at the end of each breath. Notice the gap between the end of exhaling and the beginning of inhaling. Imagine that while in the gap, you are in the presence of spirit.

❖ Since spirit is not a physical entity, you can only experience the undulations of spirit (like a ripple effect). You are no longer accessing the mind or identifying a physical area. This is a contemplative dimension that does not respond to linear thinking.

❖ Continue focusing on your breathing and repeating "Spirit" at the end of each breath. Witness the gap between breaths with a consciousness of receptivity. Do not try to control or prolong the gap; just let the process guide you.

❖ When you are in the gap, experience its boundlessness. And in that boundlessness, switch from the spirit mantra to "I am spirit."

❖ Continue repeating the "I am spirit" mantra for a few minutes, and then move on to "I am spirit wherever I go."

❖ Notice that, because of the essence of spirit, I propose "I am" for the third mantra rather than "I take." Also, if you do not believe in God or a deity, you can still use spirit to represent something more universal than yourself (for example, nature, or Buddhahood).

❖ Now you are ready for the most important step. Stop reciting the mantra, and permit yourself to trust that it continues to be expressed in your *implicate consciousness*—a dimension that is inaccessible to intellect. (I will also explain the notion of implicate consciousness in the Going Deeper section.)

❖ Shift your attention from the gap between breaths
to the gap between thoughts. Trust, without seeking
evidence, that *transcendental wisdom* resides in the
gap, and accept the experience as the most auspicious
(best fit) in the long run. The gap experience reflects
implicate wisdom rather than intelligible information.
This trusting process is the mindbody code for taking
a leap of faith. It is consciousness without form. Note
that I am not referring to religious faith here. Instead,
it is faith as a path to spiritual wisdom.

❖ When you are ready to end the exercise, count from
one to ten, open your eyes, and slowly reorient yourself
before getting up.

Notice that, whereas the first four portals have physical
dimensions in which thoughts, feelings, and sensations can
be experienced in time and space, the fifth portal is absent of
content and physicality, in time without space. Consider what
you experienced in the gap between thoughts as undulations
of spirit. Although the undulations are not easily discernible in
the early stages of this training, they are implicitly generating
beneficial, delayed effects; the wisdom inherent in the gap
unfolds when you need it rather than when you expect it. As
you become more proficient in witnessing the gap, you may
notice more instances of synchronicity in your life as well as
more lucid solutions surfacing when needed to enable you to
confront complex challenges.

◇◇

GOING DEEPER INTO THE
CONTEMPLATIVE FOUNDATION

You will find that I repeat and expand upon the biocognitive concepts I introduce in each chapter. This method of teaching is based on how the brain

learns complex information. Repetition strengthens the neuromaps that conceptualize the subject, and expansion deepens the abstractions needed to understand the subject in a variety of different contexts. Biocognition is a language that replaces or expands what you already know in another language.

The five portals exercise introduces you to the experiential dimension of the mindbody code. The technique is deceptively simple in that it incidentally equips you with a powerful compass to navigate a private journey of self that replaces the rigidity of fear with the expansiveness of discovery. The three mantras chosen for each portal provide transition from the semantic symbol (the language dimension of a word) to an embodied biosymbol (the *felt meaning* of the word).

Let me explain further: the semantic space of the portals' first mantras resides in the mind as symbols of safety, love, expression, peace, and spirit. When the symbols are personified by adding "I am" to the second mantra, the semantic space shifts from mind to *embodied mind*. Then, with the third mantra, that embodied mind accompanies you wherever you go. For example, the mantra "Love" brings awareness to the concept of love; the mantra "I am love" infuses love consciousness into the fabric of your identity; and finally, "I take love wherever I go" allows you to experience that consciousness everywhere.

In later chapters, I will introduce you to more advanced methods that transform the world of ordinary eyesight into the empowered vision of a mystical scientist—or a scientific mystic. The concepts and practical methods I offer in this book are a synthesis of biocognitive science and contemplative psychology. The former investigates how cultures shape our perception, and the latter studies the psychology of different theologies. Together they give us a formula to explore mind-body-spirit with proven Western and Eastern methodologies.

Pairing the biosymbols of safety, love, expression, and peace with physical portals exposes you to the experiential language of the mindbody code. The exercise to acquaint you with the spiritual portal and learn to navigate implicate consciousness expands the experiential language of the mindbody code to the transcendental dimension of self. In the biocognitive paradigm, we approach mind-body-spirit as an inseparable entity that seeks wisdom and asserts wellness as a birthright.

Now, as I promised earlier, I will say a bit more about the two essential concepts I introduced in this first experiential exercise.

Undulations of Spirit

Teresa of Avila and other mystical theologians, as well as Søren Kierkegaard and other existential philosophers, explain that, because of the physical limitations of our faculties, we cannot access spirit directly. Instead, spirit is invited with a leap of faith. The technique you learned for the fifth portal is one of the transcendental pathways to experiencing the undulations (the ripple aftereffects) of a nonphysical process: awareness without context.

Implicate Consciousness

This is the collective knowledge that surfaces into awareness based on the demands of cultural contexts. Consciousness is bound by beliefs that have horizons that determine the edge of awareness. We can only perceive what we believe exists, but because of our implicate consciousness, we know more than we can explain.

THERAPEUTIC BENEFITS OF THE FIVE PORTALS TECHNIQUE

The five portals technique has several therapeutic benefits. First, it teaches you to identify where you manifest stress in your body and the biosymbols that you associate with the stressors. In other words, it allows you to identify biosymbolic patterns and the conditions (cultural contexts) that trigger each portal. For instance, do you experience stress in one portal more frequently than in another one? Do you find unique situations that trigger a particular portal over another (for example, safety rather than love)? As you make connections between stressful conditions and mindbody-spirit manifestations, you can use the witnessing and breathing method to soothe the affected portal.

Another benefit is that attention without interpretation—or witnessing—accesses the mindbody code that relieves physical tension and emotional anguish. It is a method of healing with mindfulness. Research in psychoneuroimmunology and contemplative psychology shows that the simple action of focusing attention on an affected area can reduce pain and inflammation there, accelerate wound healing, stabilize heart rhythm, and increase brain wave coherence, and has many other beneficial biocognitive effects.

Identifying the five portals of wellness in yourself and recognizing your unique expression of dissonance in each of the portals unfolds the mindbody cultural history you have assimilated. For each portal, you have identified what your culture taught you to inhibit, where the tension manifests in your mindbody, and how to punish your transgressions. Now that you are gaining a holistic view of how you live your cultural admonitions, you can relinquish what does not serve you well and engage the *causes* of health I will teach you to identify. You will learn much more about what causes a state of health as you journey through the book.

❖ ❖ ❖

In the next chapter, I will introduce you to archetypal wounds—wounds that all cultures around the globe inflict upon their people. And I will teach you how to access the healing fields to resolve these wounds.

Archetypal Wounds
and Their Healing Fields

All cultures, East and West, have their own unique ways of punishing those whose ideas and behaviors run contrary to established beliefs. These forms of punishment cause emotional damage that surfaces in the form of three *archetypal wounds:* abandonment, shame, and betrayal. I call these wounds archetypal because they are so remarkably consistent across cultures—and the similarities in their mindbody manifestations are striking. It was seeing the detrimental effects that such wounds had on the health and well-being of my patients that moved me to find "antidotes" to reverse the damage. And now I will share them with you.

I discovered something profound. There is a healing field for each of the three wounds. *Commitment* heals abandonment, *honor* heals shame, and *loyalty* heals betrayal. I will teach you to access and work with these three healing fields.

BIOINFORMATIONAL FIELDS

In biocognitive theory, a *field* is an expression of the mindbody that cannot be separated from its cultural interpretation. *Bioinformation* itself is the full cultural meaning contained within a field. For example, in Western cultures, the bioinformational field for the way we greet one another—the *greeting field*—includes shaking hands. In some Middle Eastern cultures, the greeting field involves placing a hand over the heart. So each culture expresses a greeting based on its cultural history. Although each culture determines the conditions that constitute a greeting field, or any other field, I have found that the mindbody responses to that field are very similar across cultures.

Cultures also have differences in *rites of passage fields*. In Spain, the rite of passage field for adolescent boys involves making the local soccer team, while for the Masai tribe of East Africa, it may require defending their herd from a lion attack. What is common to both cultures is that a boy can be shamed for failing at his rite of passage. In these two instances, the requirements for passage could hardly be more culturally different, but the boy who does not make the soccer team and the boy who fails to slay the lion will both experience the archetypal wound of shame. This wound will manifest in their bodies in predictable ways, with specific responses on the part of the immune, nervous, and endocrine systems. In the next chapter, I will explain how these biological systems respond to deprecating emotions, but for now the important point is this: each archetypal wound constitutes its own *wounding field* and has unique emotional patterns that, when allowed to become a way of life, can detract from wellness and trigger illness.

LEARNING THE LANGUAGE OF WOUNDS

We acquire archetypal wounds gradually and in a language that is actually a form of control. Parents, teachers, and other authority figures act as cultural editors and use the language of shame, abandonment, and betrayal to punish us when we violate our culture's established beliefs or behaviors. If you were consistently shamed when you deviated from what your parents, teachers, or other cultural editors expected of you, you inadvertently learned to "speak" shame fluently. Why? Because our cultural editors are important to us; they are people we love, need, respect, or fear—and may even be all of these combined. They play important roles in molding our self-concept. In the process of loving us or protecting us, their attempts to control our digressions also wound us.

In fact, in order to be accepted by the cultural editors we loved and needed in our youth, we had to submit our mistakes and digressions to them for review: a less than stellar report card from school, or a failed attempt to sit still at the dinner table. And in their subsequent wounding of us, they justified their punishments with statements such as "I am doing this for your own good."

This is how we learned an intimate language that entangles love and wounds. Gradually, we learned to use that intimate language to control ourselves and others, and later in life, we will allow others to shame, abandon, or betray us because we think they, too, are doing us a favor. It works the other way around as well; we will wound others, believing that we are doing it for their benefit.

We always have the option of blaming the cultural editors of our past for our current distress—and thereby remain in distress. But there is a better way. We can instead untangle the communication pattern that links love with shame, abandonment, or betrayal. We can do this by engaging the healing field that corresponds to the wound: engaging honor for the pain of shame, commitment for the pain of abandonment, and loyalty for the pain of betrayal.

For example, if you were wounded by shame as a child, as an adult today, it is very possible to consciously create for yourself living conditions that are based on honor. It is important to understand that this process is three-pronged: it involves awareness of all three types of wounds and their healing fields. While healing shame (through its antidote, honor) may be your main goal at this point in your life, you can create the conditions of honor that will heal shame without betraying the commitment (the antidote to abandonment) you have made to heal your shame. So you can see that all three fields are related and can work together to help you heal your deep archetypal wounds. In later chapters, I'll have more to say about using all three healing fields concurrently.

A Gradual Approach

I recommend you incorporate all these new biocognitive concepts gradually—you need not rush. In order to achieve sustainable change, you have to *confront, release,* and *replace* what you intend to modify, and this takes time. It entails confronting your fears, releasing a dysfunction that has become a way of life for you, and replacing the sense of unworthiness you feel, which conjures obstacles to improving your quality of life, with worthiness. You cannot work through all of these layers at the snap of a finger. But if you use the right tools to approach a dysfunctional pattern, over time your fears will crumble, and your sense of self-worth will grow. All the while, your focus is on the process of change itself—the journey toward change—not on the end goal.

AGENTS OF SUSTAINABLE CHANGE

Most of us know why we need to change, but achieving actual transformation can be an overwhelming task when we focus on just part of the bioinformational field we are trying to change. Reasoning, for example, encompasses only the mind's contribution to the bioinformational field, and emotions reflect only what the body experiences. Working with just one excludes the other. And working with both, reasoning and emotions together, still doesn't address the cultural conditions that contextualized the learned patterns—placed them in the context of your culture—in the first place. We need to work with all three components, the mind, the body, and the cultural context, to create change that lasts.

Are you finding any of the discussion so far confusing? If you are, congratulations! You have just accessed the first agent of change: *turbulence.* The turbulence you are experiencing increases instability at the horizons of the bioinformational field, and this instability gives you the opportunity to assimilate or reject new information.

To further explain, the bioinformational field is contained by a fluid edge rather than a rigid boundary; it is amenable to change. But when you fear the turbulence of change, the horizon loses its fluidity, becoming an inflexible constraint upon your ability to change. Lasting change requires this "shaking up" stage to recontextualize (re-envision) the functional meaning that has been supporting a behavior you want to change.

For example, modifying our habits of addiction, obsession, or compulsion affects whichever dysfunction is involved, but it does not change the contextual mindbody meaning that sustains the dysfunction.

Where addictions are concerned, in addition to any genetic predisposition we may have, the functional meaning that underlies addictive behavior is *self-destructive distraction to avoid feeling worthy*. We relinquished this sense of worthiness when we experienced our archetypal wounds. But why in the world would we want to avoid regaining our worthiness—why distract ourselves from this prospect? Because, just as supportive love teaches us that we are valuable and worthy of a good life, archetypal wounds teach us to devalue who we are and believe that we are unworthy of a good life. We invest in confirming what our cultural editors have taught us to believe, rather than what we have the potential to become.

For instance, if you believe that poverty is your destiny, any condition that challenges that belief will cause turbulence for you; it will make you very uncomfortable. This explains a phenomenon that would otherwise remain a great mystery: the fact that people in the United States who win huge sums of money in the lottery lose it within an average of eighteen months. If we do not feel worthy of it, even good fortune can become our worst enemy.

Similarly, many rehab programs fail because they focus on changing the addictive behavior rather than on the distraction from one's intrinsic self-worth that the addictive behavior provides. Fear-, anger-, and guilt-based approaches to modifying a behavior fail miserably because they are irreconcilable with the agents of sustainable change; fear induces avoidance, anger invites aggression, and guilt promotes punishment. While some negative emotions can trigger a need for and inspire change, they mostly wound instead.

Now I'm going to expand your newly fluid horizons further by introducing you to two more important terms in biocognition. The true agents of change are *elevated cognitions* and *exalted emotions*. These agents of change provide sustained transformation; in fact, they have triumphed over the greatest infamies and darkest periods in our human journey.

Elevated cognitions could be considered "higher thinking." These include such thoughts as admiration, recognition of moral conduct, dignity, modesty, and other concepts that reflect graceful acknowledgment of human excellence, in self and others. *Exalted emotions* encompass love, empathy, compassion, gratitude, awe, inspiration, and any other feeling that confirms that which is noble in self and others.

These two agents of sustainable change are extremely powerful. They have facilitated the mindbody cultural conditions responsible for bringing an end to slavery, genocide, prejudice, hegemony, and other atrocities that plague humanity in the name of religion or idealism. That is how strong they are. I characterize them both as *laudable fields*. If they have been powerful enough to overcome tyranny, we can safely conclude that they are equally effective when applied to individual change. We can apply the same *dignity field* that ended apartheid to ending smoking, overeating, or any other self-destructive conduct that lacks *inclusive compassion,* a concept in Tibetan Buddhist psychology that views compassion for self as inseparable from compassion toward others. The collective wounding field of shame that maintained apartheid in South Africa (with the ruling whites degrading the blacks) was resolved with the healing field of honor that brought racial equality and an end to infamy.

However, changing any dysfunctional condition leaves a vacuum. So, just as Nelson Mandela prevented a bloodbath of revenge when he created the Truth and Reconciliation Commission (which commuted or reduced sentences for government officials who admitted their crimes), we must fill the vacuum with choices that inspire sustainable improvement.

So it is that the healing fields of honor, commitment, and loyalty can heal the archetypal wounds of shame, abandonment, and betrayal that obstruct our attempts to reach personal excellence.

UNMASKING AVOIDANCE

Moving now from the conceptual to the practical, let's begin to decipher the mechanisms that are at work when we fail to change a dysfunctional behavior, despite knowing that change is in our best interest. If we can see the behavior we are trying to change as an act of avoidance, we can (1) identify the wound that we are reluctant to confront and (2) identify the healing field we lack the feelings of self-worth to embrace. We can also identify what condition we can create to replace the vacuum that may be left by the absence of the destructive behavior we've been engaging in. We must do this *before* we implement the change that is going to create the vacuum.

Although we may be aware of the discomfort we feel from dysfunction today, the emotional investment we have made in our dysfunctional behavior originally served us well as a distraction from painful wounds. Since any investment, be it in something with positive or negative impacts, creates attachments, one of the paths to freedom from painful conditions is to mourn the end of our attachment to known misery. As we learn to confront the true causes of our discomfort (our archetypal wounds), redefine their cultural contexts, and embrace their healing fields, we must also mourn the end of a familiar if harmful companionship—our avoidance mechanism. Only then can we fill that vacuum with the dignity fields that have long bested the darkest side of our human tribal journeys.

It is important to note that certain unwanted actions that are not necessarily related to wounds can also become habitual. We can certainly learn inefficient ways of behaving that, through repetition, become habits that are disconnected from our awareness. For example, we may habitually take a long, congested road to work, and fail to notice how frustrated we are when we reach our destination. But once we pay attention to how we feel, we can consider alternative routes. In fact, these kinds of discoveries can bring great joy when they lift a burden we have created through simple lack of awareness rather than by avoiding wounds.

PATHS TO KNOWLEDGE

Some biocognitive teaching methods may appear counterintuitive, but they offer practical alternatives to the conventional life sciences' view of human beings as biochemical machines. Learning the experiential mindset will help you understand why some highly intelligent people can make profoundly unwise decisions, why some self-proclaimed gurus lead miserable lives, and why pharmaceutical companies invest fortunes in formulating medications for relief of symptoms rather than cures. All of these paradoxes are the result of a reductionist thinking that leaves out cultural contexts and fails to recognize that *reasoning* is not the same as *embodying*.

Conventional biology borrowed from reductionist Newtonian physics what is called *upward causality*, going from the simplest to the most complex mechanics of a system. For example, if a car is leaking gas, the solution is to fix the leak, whether the car is in Paris or the Brazilian Amazon. It works! But if we generalize reductionist solutions to human beings, they frequently fail. Why? Because the complexity of living systems, including human beings, is neither reducible to its functions nor independent of contextual conditions. In other words, unlike machines, we give meaning to our actions within cultural contexts.

If a person of European ancestry living in New York City is diagnosed with anemia, a physician can treat it successfully. But if the same symptoms of anemia (fatigue, shortness of breath, dizziness) are diagnosed in an Indian or mestizo patient by an Aymara shaman in the Bolivian Andes as *limpu*, no amount of intervention by Western medicine can save the patient. The cause of limpu is culturally attributed to witnessing a stillbirth, and the belief is that the spirit of the infant consumes the body of the person who witnessed it so the spirit can remain on earth. Interestingly, white Bolivians living in that exact same area of the Andes do not succumb to limpu because their Western cultural ancestry does not contextualize anemia as limpu. This is a striking example of the myriad ways in which our biological functioning is strongly influenced by the cultural attributions we give to causes of illness. Similarly, if when you were a child your mother told you not to go out in rain because you'll catch a cold, that warning—coming as it does from an important authority figure—is likely to become prophesy.

Although I will fully explain *embodied perception* using scientific evidence in the next chapter, here I will first introduce the concept of *embodiment*. According to biocognitive theory, "knowing" is more than rationally understanding information. This is why trying to reason our way out of unwanted behavior has such limited success. It's like trying to help an addict by simply explaining that the abused substance is dangerous, solving your chronic hostility by recognizing that it can lead to cardiovascular disorders, or coming out of a depression by deciding to think happy thoughts. None of these scenarios is realistic. So why does changing the dysfunctional behaviors that can harm us require much more than intellectual appeal? Here is where embodiment can provide some of the answers.

Perception is accomplished by mindbody actions in time and space. If there is no action, the senses involved cannot assimilate the associations the brain makes about an event. But the brain makes its interpretations in *coauthorship* with the body. We perceive with a mindbody process that cannot be separated from the cultural context in which the perception takes place. If you find a lion in your living room, your mindbody reaction will be very different than if you see that same lion at the circus. Thus, embodiment is the mindbody *incorporation* of what we perceive. The word "incorporate" comes from the Latin *incorporatus,* united into one body. Although we embody what we perceive, we seem to function as if intellect (the mind) were the only agent involved.

Now let's further clarify those heavy explanations of embodied perception with practical examples. We are *embodying* when we walk the walk rather than talk the talk, when we *feel* the meaning of a word, when we experience the profoundness of love, when we are engulfed in an act of compassion, when we feel facial tension the moment we notice we are frowning. The crux of the matter is this: we learn *embodied* dysfunctions, and we hopelessly attempt to change them with *disembodied* reasoning. Let's celebrate the insight that resistance to change has less to do with intellect than with lacking the proper experiential tools. Imagine how well even a genius could drive a nail using a screwdriver instead of a hammer.

HEALING FROM WITHIN

We should not dismiss the contributions of modern medical science. While imagery, attribution, and hope can be powerful healing agents when applied in the appropriate contexts, using imagery alone to reset a compound fracture would be ineffective; attributing an internal bleeding condition to bad luck would ignore the real cause; and merely hoping that the islets of Langerhans will generate beta cells in a person with insulin-dependent diabetes would only lead to profound disappointment. Nonetheless, although they are infrequent, spontaneous remissions (instant healing) of terminal illnesses persistently baffle the biological sciences because their mechanistic model of life does not accommodate conditions that so radically defy "established" prognoses. Paradoxically, the imagery, attribution, and hope that I just discouraged us from relying upon in the face of certain medical conditions can be powerful healing agents when applied in the appropriate contexts. We need to fuse the best of modern integrative medicine with the wisdom of mindbody science to create a joint path to healing.

There are several reasons why reductionist medicine denies that mindbody processes have any therapeutic value.

* Reductionist medicine intervenes with its mechanical model only *after* there is physical evidence of illness; what we can't see yet does not exist.
* Alternative therapies have not consistently submitted their methods to rigorous scientific evaluation; we need scientific evidence before we can believe.
* Just as reductionist medicine underestimates the contributions of the mind in the healing process, alternative therapies tend to overestimate what the mind can do independent of the body; it's either mind or body.

What can we do to help these two extreme positions find wisdom in a middle way and incorporate their proven contributions? We can explore what causes health. In doing so, we can incorporate (embody) the best contributions of each discipline, discard the predatory and obstinate elements of both, and commit to advancing our knowledge of how the beliefs we embody (the philosophies we live) from our cultural histories can affect gene expression and promote mindbody healing processes. The industries that profit by reducing our humanity to biochemical and mechanical parts disdain such concepts. I submit this means we must be on to something.

PUTTING THE THEORIES TO WORK

It is time to begin to put what you have learned thus far in this chapter into practice. The following series of exercises forms the foundation for identifying and healing archetypal wounds. The process encompasses seven steps:

1 Identifying your archetypal wound(s) and the cultural editors implicated in their creation.

2 Embodying your memories of the archetypal wound(s).

3 Untangling your archetypal wounds from your *intimate language of love.*

4 Accessing your history of elevated cognitions and exalted emotions.

5 Mourning your known misery before replacing the vacuum it will leave behind.

6 Embodying the healing fields.

7 Evaluating your relationships with your present coauthors of both misery and excellence.

THE POWER OF CONTEMPLATION

You can embody each of the objectives I just listed by using contemplative methods that reduce muscle tension and quiet the internal dialogues of your mind, just as you did in your exploration of the portals of wellness at the end of chapter 1. This will allow you to access, without distractions, the mindbody memories of your archetypal wound(s). The method is called *contemplative* because it shifts awareness from *interpreting* to *witnessing* the interpretations. Rather than being the object the mind is observing, contemplation is the experience of observing the mind: noticing that it gives attention to one thing over another; that awareness shifts from thoughts to sensations to emotions; that the contents frequently shift, and so on.

By relaxing your body and reducing the internal noise of your mind, contemplation opens a direct portal to your archetypal wounds. (Note that I use the word *portal* here as I did in chapter 1, and will use it elsewhere in the book as well. I have found it the best term to describe the entryway to a bioinformational field.) The usual distractions you use to avoid confronting your wounds cannot enter the wounding fields where the symbols of shame, abandonment, and betrayal function as biosymbols. For example, the word *shame* is a symbol that represents the hurtful statements that cause the emotion of shame: "You're stupid," "You're worthless," or "You're bad." When the word *shame* is embodied, the symbol is transformed into a biosymbol that can trigger embarrassment, blushing, drooping shoulders, and other degrading mindbody manifestations. The word acquires biological properties.

The contemplative method allows uninterrupted access to the archives of your archetypal wounds so you can experience the associated biosymbols without judgment, identify how and where the mindbody effects surface in your life, and learn who the implicated cultural editors were and the approximate age you were when you received the wound. It is best to access the earliest possible incidence of a wounding to determine the level of abstraction you were capable of using when you first conceptualized the wounding event.

Your age at the time you experienced a wound determines the level of meaning you can give it when you contextualize and store it away in memory. A five-year-old interprets a wound more concretely than a fifteen-year-old because our capacities to conceptualize abstract language increase as we mature. Based on the developmental stage, interpretations could range from, "What I did wrong means I am a bad person" to "What I did wrong was a bad thing."

Before you delve into the contemplative methods that follow, remember that the mindbody code pathways are accessed indirectly and communicated experientially. They do not operate in a linear or intellectual fashion. As we have explored in this chapter, simply reasoning out or wishing for a solution does not change the conditions that maintain dysfunctional mindbody patterns. Their nonintellectual composition is the main reason why archetypal wounds cannot be healed by using logical appeal. At this point, I ask you to trust that you know more than you can intellectually explain to yourself.

<><><><><><><><><><><><><><><><><><><><><><><><><><><><><>

Identifying Archetypal Wounds and Cultural Editors

We start with relaxation. Each of the following experiential stages begins with the same contemplative method:

* Sit in a quiet place and gently close your eyes. Rather than trying to relax, control your thoughts, or engage in any other intentional action, simply observe your mindbody activity. Nonintentionality is the pathway to a contemplative experience.

* Observe the thoughts, emotions, and sensations that enter and exit your awareness.

* Allow your mindbody awareness to flow, without directing or labeling the flow.

* After about five minutes of contemplative witnessing, gently search for your earliest memories of a possible archetypal wound. When you trace the first memory of a wound, recreate the experience, the circumstances when the cultural editor(s) *taught* you the wound, and your approximate age at the time. Then drop the imagery and pay attention to how it physically manifests in your body. For example, you remember telling a lie to your mother, and she caught you in that lie. Your best guess is that you were five years old at the time. When she scolded you, you felt ashamed.

* Identify any sensations of heat or cold when the wound surfaces, the area where you sense the wounding in

your body, the emotions that surface, and your *feelings* rather than your *thoughts* about the cultural editor you have identified. For example, you feel a sensation of heat around your chest.

❖ You will note a variety of sensations when the wounds surface from memory. Abandonment feels cold, for example, while shame and betrayal feel hot. In the next chapter, I will expand on the physiological sensations associated with each wound.

❖ After a few minutes of contemplative observations, you can wind down the exercise by imagining you are watching the end of a play; someone on stage has been telling you a story of a wounding, and the curtain is now closing.

❖ To reenter a state of serenity, simply witness—without interpreting—any residual bodily tension and "mind noise." Breathe gently to prepare for the next stage.

Since the resolution of archetypal wounds does not involve reasoning, after you have experienced your wounding and identified the cultural editors involved, it is not necessary for you to try to understand what happened—there are no mind solutions for mindbody conditions. Instead you want to reach a contemplative state of noninterpretation.

<><><><><><><><><><><><><><><><><><><><><><><><>

Untangling Archetypal Wounds from the Intimate Language of Love

❖ Remaining in a quiet place, gently close your eyes again. Rather than trying to relax, control your thoughts, or engage in any other intentional action, simply observe your mindbody activity.

❖ Observe the thoughts, emotions, and sensations that enter and exit your awareness.

❖ Allow your mindbody awareness to flow, without labeling what flows.

❖ After a few minutes of contemplative witnessing, bring to awareness your archetypal wound and the cultural editor involved with the wound.

❖ Experience the wound in association with the cultural editor. Sense the love, fear, admiration, disgust, resentment, or any other emotion you may feel related to the cultural editor at the time of wounding. Observe where the sensations and emotions manifest in your body. For example, your mother's anger makes you feel afraid—you fear both punishment and rejection. You feel a clenching sensation in your belly.

This experience helps you identify the positive and negative entanglements of your intimate language of love. Because an insult to our worthiness can diminish our capacity to love, even wounds from strangers whom we never loved can indirectly compromise how we assimilate and communicate our intimate language of love. Simply put, feeling worthy is a precursor of love.

Now that you have experienced the emotions entangled with your intimate language of love, let's begin the disentanglement:

❖ Return to the contemplative state and, after a few minutes, access memories of a time when you felt compassion, empathy, gratitude, or admiration for yourself or for someone other than the cultural editor you have identified. Experience the emotions that surface, along with the warmth and connection you may feel for yourself or the other person. For example, you recall a time when you reached out to someone when you were in the waiting room of a doctor's office. You could tell that this person was very anxious, and you sat quietly beside him, believing that your calm presence might be helpful. After a minute or two, he emitted a great sigh and relaxed.

❖ Now that you have experienced feelings of love that were not entangled with deprecating wounds, you can recognize the distinctly different felt meanings of both types: *contaminated love* and pristine love.

❖ Bring back the same experiences of entangled (contaminated) love—your lie and your mother's anger—and witness its unfolding, without attempting to modify what happened at the time. Now bring back the pristine experience of unconditional love—your caring for a stranger—and witness how it unfolds, again without attempting to change anything.

❖ Now shift back and forth between experiencing memories of entangled love and experiencing memories of pristine love. Do the shifting exercise several times, and pay close attention to the shifting moments. Breathe slowly to prepare for the next experience.

This is a very powerful step because contemplatively witnessing the *shifts* is what untangles the wounds from the intimate language of love. Although the time/space between thoughts is experienced as gaps and the time/space between entangled and pristine love is experienced as shifts, profound recontextualizing can take place in what appear to be vacuums. But rather than vacuums, gaps, or shifts, the experiences are actually transitional states of mindbody processes. These states are amenable to change through contemplation but hopelessly impervious to intellectual interventions—and this is what you are after! Since you are used to functioning at a level where reason is the agent of change, it may be difficult to understand that deeper levels of transformation can take place through contemplating these apparent vacuums where nothing seems to happen. I will further describe these biocognitive concepts following this experiential section.

◇◇◇◇◇◇◇◇◇◇◇◇◇◇◇◇◇◇◇◇◇◇◇◇◇◇◇◇◇◇◇◇◇◇◇◇◇

Mourn the Known Misery
before Replacing the Vacuum

❖ After you have reached a contemplative state, shift to imagining what would happen if you could communicate using a pristine language of love. How would your relationships change? What could you accomplish? What would you do differently in your life? For example, your interactions with others would be more meaningful. You would feel like you could communicate more honestly. You would receive more love in return, and as a result, you would be more willing to make genuine contact with people more often.

❖ Pay attention, without interpreting, to what your mindbody is experiencing while you are imagining entirely new possibilities in your life.

❖ Now, identify what it is that the entangled language of love is allowing you to avoid. It may be allowing you to avoid something you fear having to do or something you would like to do.

❖ What did the entangled language of love allow you to avoid that you feared or disliked? What did it allow you to sabotage that you felt unworthy of accepting? In other words, the damage that wounds can inflict on your sense of self-worth can paradoxically lead you to sabotage your own attempts to correct your failures as well as your attempts to succeed in life. For example, "Tangling love and shame allows me to avoid genuine contact so I don't risk rejection or judgment."

❖ Experience the mindbody manifestations that arise when you imagine confronting whatever it is that you have avoided out of fear. After a few minutes, shift to imagining what you have avoided out of a lack of self-worth, and experience the related mindbody manifestations. Experience this shifting for a few more minutes, and detach from the experience. For example, you have an opportunity to apply for a position at work that has prestige and a higher salary, but you find a way to avoid it because you lack the self-worth to accept the promotion that comes your way.

After you begin to heal your archetypal wounds, approaching what you have avoided because of fear and feelings of unworthiness offers the ingredients that will fill the vacuum.

◇◇◇

Embodying the Healing Fields

A reminder: honor heals shame, commitment heals abandonment, and loyalty heals betrayal. Just as we all have memories of being shamed, abandoned, or betrayed, we also have memories of our moments of honor, commitment, and loyalty. Although insults to our sense of self-worth can erode our memories of our more laudable conduct, biocognitive contemplations can resurrect the elevated thoughts and exalted emotions we have neglected, heal our wounds, and free us from self-deprecation.

❖ After you have reached a contemplative state, shift to recalling early memories of experiences that you can relate to the healing field that corresponds with your archetypal wound. For example, if you were wounded with shame, you would imagine memories of honorable moments in your life, such as remembering having stood up for a classmate who was being made fun of in the school yard at recess. You were a little afraid, but knew what the other kids were doing wasn't right. You got them to back down.

❖ Bring back other memories of worthy conduct related to your healing field, and experience your mindbody manifestations. Shift from these memories to other laudable examples from memory, and experience the shifting moments.

❖ Once you have established an experiential foundation where you can clearly identify with your worthy memories, begin shifting from memories of your archetypal wound to memories of your healing fields. Pay close attention to the gaps and shifts between memories.

❖ Notice how the shifting begins to affect the quality of your opposing memories. The *healing field* gains strength while the *archetypal wound field* dissipates. Continue the shifting process for a few more minutes, and then return to serenity. Give yourself a few minutes to become reoriented before getting up.

◇◇

Evaluating Our Relationships with Our Coauthors of Misery and Joy

As a final step in this process, you will take a look at the coauthors of your present life and consider whether different actions on your part might better support you in sustaining the changes you wish to see.

❖ Identify any coauthors in your family or social circles who communicate a kind of helplessness that supports victimhood. For example, your cousin hates his job but he never looks for anything better. He says there's too much competition out there, and he's probably in the best situation he would be able to find.

❖ Rather than trying to change these detracting coauthors, decide how much contact you want to have with them and the quality of that contact. If they are hopelessly committed to misery, you may have to break off contact altogether. If you choose not to end a negative relationship, then limit the level of love you can share without taking on any toxicity. For example, you love your cousin, but being with him sometimes seems to sap your energy. Maybe you'll limit your contact with him to accompanying him to sporting events, when he seems to lighten up.

❖ Identify coauthors in your family or social circles who enhance your worthiness. Determine whether you may be neglecting them or taking them for granted. Celebrate with them the simple moments in life that are taken for granted. For example, your good friend always seems to mention something she likes or admires about you, even if it's just what you're wearing, or a small thing you accomplished recently. It's high time you went out for coffee again.

❖ Rather than trying to change any of your coauthors, change your responses to them. Understand that if you choose to maintain a relationship with someone out of guilt or fear, the weight of that relationship's toxicity will only increase.

◇◇

WHAT MAKES THESE METHODS WORK

Did you notice that the healing fields themselves have no connection at all to whoever initially perpetrated the wound? Did you wonder why? Did you notice that you can feel the healing symbols (words) when you embody them? Did you experience any difficulties in shifting from interpreting with the mind to contemplating the mind's actions?

After years of searching for methods that give us access to our biosymbolic wounds, and then offering opportunities to heal them, I discovered that any such interventions had to be experiential. The wounds have been archived in fields of biosymbolic meaning, and the solutions are hidden in the gaps and shifts between thoughts, feelings, and sensations in our stream of consciousness. These apparent *segments of nothingness* between fields of experience are far from empty or meaningless. Rather than containing substance, the segments of nothingness represent moments in time and space when a mindbody field has the highest probability of recontextualizing its biosymbolic meaning: a change in the mindbody meaning of a context that offers space for healing to take place.

For another way to think about what I am proposing, imagine a mindbody field as a coherent unit of knowledge that contains all the information necessary to find meaning in a concept, belief, emotion, memory, or sensation. In the case of an archetypal wound, the field would contain the thoughts, emotions, and sensations that make up the total experience of the wound. Now imagine that these fields are held inside containers that have flexible horizons rather than rigid boundaries; their horizons are permeable, flexible, and variable. This allows information exchange and new learning to take place between fields. But if new learning (change) is painful, fear can block access to these flexible horizons.

In the process of contemplatively witnessing the mind's stream of consciousness, we notice the gaps and shifts that we fail to experience when we are actively thinking and going about our business. In the contemplative state of observation, what appear to be segments of nothingness are actually horizons between fields of meaningful information! Since the horizons are the most variable condition of a field, they are where the highest probability for new learning is likeliest to take place. During the contemplative experience, without obstructions from our fears, profound change can take place at these horizons.

But how can simply witnessing these horizons accomplish change? Because, with the *biocognitive contemplative method,* we can witness a field horizon (for example, shame) and *shift* to witnessing another field horizon (for example, honor), alternating from one field to the other. The shifting of fields allows an opportunity for a *meeting of horizons.*

In other words, we create a condition in which biosymbolic meaning can change. And here is one of the most important principles in biocognitive theory: *our elevated cognitions and exalted emotions have greater capacity to shift biosymbolic meaning than do our more primal thoughts and feelings.* The former grow with love while the latter are impeded by fear. Consequently, if we allow a meeting of horizons between the healing and wounding fields, because healing fields are vastly more powerful, honor will inevitably overwhelm shame, commitment will resolve abandonment, and loyalty will transcend betrayal.

Even more important, this method works because, rather than attempt to change our memories of the cultural editors who wounded us, we allow ourselves to recontextualize (change the felt meaning of) the helplessness that the wound created. And here is a critical concept to grasp if we are to understand the healing mechanism at work: *a wound is a state of helplessness, and healing is a return to empowerment.*

Years of clinical experience working with people who have the most traumatic of histories have taught me to approach complex conditions with interventions—such as you have just experienced—that draw power from their simplicity and elegance. Repetition is required, and I invite you to continue your biocognitive journey as if you were learning a new language. As with learning a new language, you must practice, and apply what you have learned to new experiences as they arise.

❖ ❖ ❖

In the next chapter, we will explore the mindbody relationship with the nervous, immune, and endocrine systems, and I will introduce scientific evidence to support my argument that cultural beliefs have greater influence on our health than does our genetic endowment. The material is technical, but rest assured, you will not need a background in science to understand and benefit from the information. I encourage you to explore.

Does the Immune System Have Morals?

This chapter is about the scientific foundation of biocognition. Unlike the rest of this book, which contains a sequence of concepts designed to help you learn the language of the mindbody code, this chapter is self-contained. Even if you are not technically inclined, you may find fascinating the research in mindbody communication, and it may challenge everything you were taught about health and longevity.

MINDBODY SCIENCE

Neuroscientific research has mostly focused on how the brain behaves when it has been damaged. Consequently, we have extensive knowledge of how pathology and trauma to specific areas of the brain affect behavior, but much less is known about what the brain can achieve when it's healthy. This reductionist approach limits our understanding of the complexity and plasticity of the healthy brain.

Recent studies of Tibetan monks, who are highly skilled in contemplative practices, are giving us a new understanding of how the mind can modify the chemistry, neuromapping, and structure of the brain. Some of these findings offer *adaptive* rather than pathological interpretations of mild forms of autism, attention deficit disorders, addictions, and other behaviors that are typically thought of as genetic. This means that what we thought were "illnesses" are actually adaptations to the complexities of modern life.

Not all scientists agree with these findings, however. Unfortunately, many continue to medicalize behavioral patterns of adaptation they don't understand. For example, what I call "abundance of curiosity" most health professionals diagnose as "attention deficit disorder." But before getting into controversial issues such as these, let's start with the basic principles of mindbody science.

Psychoneuroimmunology

In the 1930s, Hans Selye coined the word *stress* when his research with rats showed that threatening conditions cause hormone secretions that damage organ tissue. He borrowed the word from engineering, where stress is defined as the amount of strain a material can endure before it becomes damaged. There is no translation for the word *stress* in any language. The closest Chinese word is written with two characters: one represents "danger" and the other "opportunity," to signify "crisis."

After Selye's discovery, research continued into how stress hormones are released and affect health, but the question of mindbody communication remained speculative until thirty years later when my mentor, Dr. George F. Solomon, found that thoughts and emotions can influence the immune system. He initially studied women diagnosed with rheumatoid arthritis, an inflammatory autoimmune illness affecting women more than men, and showed that the rheumatoid factor (genetic marker) was not the only cause of the illness. In fact, he found women without the genetically determined factor who developed the illness, and others with the factor who did not. Most of the women had a history of shaming trauma, and independent of the rheumatoid factor, the ones who could identify their anger toward its perpetrator were less likely to develop the illness. *Righteous anger,* we now know, is one of the causes of health. (I will have more to say about this in other chapters.)

In addition to his stellar contributions to our understanding of autoimmune illnesses, Solomon also pioneered research into post-traumatic stress disorders, AIDS, and forensic psychiatry.

Solomon called this new, interdisciplinary science *psychoimmunology.* Approximately ten years later, Robert Ader showed that the nervous system is also involved in the intercommunication between mind and body, and renamed the field *psychoneuroimmunology* (PNI). We now know that the endocrine system is also involved, and some venture to call it *psychoneuroimmunoendocrinology.* Thus we have a piecemeal progression of terminology I have dubbed the *Frankenstein effect.* I remember phoning Solomon one day to tell him I had a new word for PNI. He asked me, "How long is it?" When I told him *biocognition* was the word, he laughed and said he thought it wasn't too bad.

In 2000, a year before he passed away, we went to Cuba together to teach a minicourse in PNI to the medical faculty at the University of Santiago de Cuba. When we arrived in the classroom, all the professors lined up to greet Solomon; the men hugged him and the women kissed him. He looked at me and said, "I was never loved like this at UCLA." I share these stories with you because I loved him like a father and still can't talk about him without tears in my eyes.

The Stress Axis

When we experience a stressful condition, although the process is complex and is not limited to the brain, the hypothalamus secretes corticotropin releasing hormones (CRH) to the pituitary, which then releases adrenocorticotropic hormone (ACTH) to the adrenal glands, which in turn release cortisol (C). This chain of hormonal secretion is called the *HPA axis* to describe the three glands involved: the hypothalamus and the pituitary are single glands in the brain, and the adrenals are a pair, located on top of the kidneys. You can appreciate, then, the traveling distance involved just to signal that something is threatening you. But if that were the only alarm system we had, it would not be fast enough to trigger the fight-or-flight response needed to confront or run from a predator. The lightning speed required to avoid a falling tree or a head-on collision is possible because of your *sympathetic nervous system,* which sends express signals from your brain to your nervous system and connects everywhere from head to toes. I will go into practical details later, but for now, it is worth taking a moment to simply appreciate the protective wisdom within you that took more than a million years to reach its present state of near perfection.

But what happens when the danger is over? On the HPA axis side, cortisol has several functions, but in the fight-or-flight response, its job is to suppress the immune system. Why? Because taking care of dangerous business is more important than fighting pathogens. So when the danger is over, *if* you are able to let go and relax, the excess cortisol signals the hypothalamus to stop the HPA hormone cascade. (I will explain later what happens when you don't let go.)

The sympathetic nervous system's fast track has a different mechanism to turn off the stress alarm. When it receives a danger signal, it increases heart rate, muscle response, blood pressure, and other systems to put you on hyperalarm; but just as important, it slows down or stops your digestion and sends blood from the stomach to your extremities so you can punch or run away. Thus, the fight-or-flight response takes precedence over fighting pathogens and digesting food (protect first, and repair and nourish later). But just like the HPA axis, the sympathetic nervous system has a mechanism to bring your body back to baseline after the danger is over. Here, the *parasympathetic nervous system* comes to the rescue and reverses the process; it slows everything down and speeds up digestion. Now your body can fight pathogens again and digest what you ate. This is why consistently taking your laptop or cell phone to meals is one of the ways you can teach your body to create digestive problems. You're telling your parasympathetic system it's time to eat, and at the same time, instructing your sympathetic system to react to your text messages or concentrated work on your laptop. This is one of the reasons why 75 percent of "busy" executives have gastrointestinal disorders. Most illnesses are learned.

Just as neuroscience has been limited by its emphasis on damaged brains, until recently psychoneuroimmunology focused most of its investigations on the effects of stress and negative emotions. I'll discuss further along in the book how the exalted emotions you first encountered in chapter 2 (love, empathy, compassion, honor, and magnanimity) affect relationships, health, and longevity. Additionally, I will propose a new model of the immune system that explains why these exalted emotions can enhance immune function, although they're unrelated to fighting pathogens.

The Neuroscience of Healthy Brains

Before we had scanning instruments like computerized tomography (CT), magnetic resonance imaging (MRI), and positron emission tomography (PET), we could only study the brain by opening the cranium after there was damage, or using the electroencephalogram (EEG), which can only provide information about the surface of the brain (the cortex). Now, not only can we see all the brain without having to open it, but thanks to functional magnetic resonance imaging (fMRI), we can also see what is going on with the brain while it's happening—activity in real time. The other scanning instruments took pictures, but with fMRI, it's like videotaping the inside of the brain.

But what is most remarkable about fMRI is that it allows us to view what the brain is doing during meditation and other contemplative practices. For example, it shows that meditation can shift brain activity from the right prefrontal lobe to the left. Why is that significant? Because when people are clinically depressed, they show more activity on the right prefrontal lobe of the brain than the left. And when antidepressants begin to work after a few weeks, there is a shift from right to left prefrontal lobes, just as when meditating. I should caution that this finding does not mean you should stop taking antidepressant medication without your doctor's advice. The fMRI studies were done with Tibetan lamas who had each practiced meditation for more than ten thousand hours. Nevertheless, if you have a physician who is a scientist rather than a technician, and who agrees to monitor your progress, you can learn meditation methods that have beneficial effects on depression without having to go live in a cave for several years.

Dr. Richard Davidson is one of the leading neuroscientists who use fMRIs to study healthy brains. His research shows something very different from what I learned when studying sick brains during my training in clinical neuropsychology. For example, the fusiform gyrus, an area close to the underside of the brain, has to do with recognizing familiar faces. But when we study the healthy brain, we find it also recognizes things we love and do well (an orchid for a florist, a rare stamp for a collector, and so on). More important, it identifies a range of functions we cannot detect when we study the damaged brain.

Let's look at what happens when we can see a range of functions versus only one. The amygdala is an almond-shaped structure, and there is one on each side of the brain. They are part of the limbic system and are responsible for signaling fear and danger. When they're damaged, you are unable to identify fear and anger in yourself and others. For example, rats with damaged amygdalae don't run away from their predators because they fail to register danger. Children with Asperger syndrome, a mild form of autism, avoid looking at others in the eyes. This limits the learning of social cues that other children gradually learn to differentiate: recognizing when people are annoyed, frustrated, tired, or experiencing other emotions by looking at telltale expressions around the eyes. Da Vinci cleverly challenged us to define Mona Lisa's smile by painting her with an ambiguous expression in her eyes. In fact, art historians have written dissertations variously arguing that it's a smile of pregnancy, betrayal, secrecy, and other creative interpretations.

Using fMRI to study healthy brains, Davidson noticed an interesting connection between the amygdala and the fusiform gyrus. He tested subjects with healthy brains and found that, when they looked at pictures that induced fear, the amygdalae lit up and the fusiform gyrus turned off; the brain was signaling to look away. When he tested children with Asperger syndrome, he found they saw the eyes as danger signals; when they looked at pictures of faces and glanced at the eyes, their amygdalae were activated, which compelled them to look away.

If we take a pathology approach to Davidson's findings, we conclude that Asperger is caused by a malfunction of the fusiform gyrus—a reductionist interpretation rather than mindbody science. But let's find out what the science I am proposing can offer instead. Davidson surmised that what appears to be malfunctioning of the fusiform gyrus in children with Asperger is actually an underdevelopment resulting from the amygdala not allowing them to learn social cues. Using fMRI to monitor, he taught a child with Asperger to turn down the amygdala and turn up the fusiform gyrus by gradually having him look at pictures of eyes that had pleasant images around them.

This approach to neuroscience is one of the foundations of the bio-cognitive tools I teach throughout this book.

Cultural Neuroscience

Biocognition places great importance on how culture shapes perception. Fortunately, *cultural neuroscience* studies how sociocultural learning influences the brain. It challenges the premise that brain function does not vary across cultures. When neuroscientists from the reductionist camp find differences in brain performance between Western and Eastern cultures, they conclude that the cause is genetic. And although they know better, this is analogous to saying there are Western and Eastern genes. Just as research on healthy brains is debunking the pathology model of the brain, cultural neuroscience is showing that cultural beliefs influence brain function.

We know that the middle area of the prefrontal lobe (above the eyebrows) formulates the concept of self-identity. Western cultures have a more individualistic conception of self than East Asian cultures, which have a more collective sense of self. Cultural neuroscientists wanted to know if these differences were reflected in the brain. When Western subjects were given tasks related to self-identity, their mid-prefrontal lobe was activated, and when they shifted to mother-related identity, it was not. But when scientists tested other cultures, they found something very different. For example, when East Asians were given the same tasks, their mid-prefrontal lobes were activated with both self *and* mother-identity. Why? Because East Asians place more importance on family interrelations than self-identity, and their brains adjust to their cultural conceptualizations.

If you took an introductory psychology course in high school or college, you may remember the Müller-Lyer optical illusion. Two parallel lines of equal length, one line with an arrow head on each end and the other with arrow tails, trick your eyes into seeing the line with two arrow tails as longer than the other. This optical illusion was considered universal until dwellers of the Kalahari Desert in southern Africa were given the test. Not affected by the optical illusion, they saw equal length when they compared the two parallel lines. By the way, other studies show that many other "optical illusions" are culturally learned as well.

I hope you can begin to appreciate why biocognition is a science of mind-body-culture. As you progress through the book you will also see why I will remove the hyphens from these three words to accentuate their inseparable composition.

CULTURAL AGING

According to biocognitive theory, longevity is mostly learned. In chapter 5, I'll share what I learned about longevity from my research with centenarians (a hundred years and older), but for now I'll continue with additional evidence to support my claim that most of our aging is culturally learned.

Research in cultural neuroscience indicates that when they perceive their respective environments, Westerners attend more to objects and East Asians to backgrounds. This indicates that Westerners place more emphasis on the figure, and East Asians on the relationship between figure and background. Memory tests confirm the cognitive differences in their visual processing, and fMRIs identify the areas of the brain that are activated. In other words, Westerners recall more objects in memory tests, and East Asians more backgrounds.

Now let's look at how aging affects this perceptual difference in visual processing. Research using fMRI demonstrates that focusing on objects activates the lateral occipital region of the brain (back of the head), and focusing on backgrounds activates the parahippocampal gyrus (part of the limbic system). When Western and East Asian subjects view pictures, Westerners activate their lateral occipital region (object preference), and the East Asians activate their parahippocampal gyrus (background preference). Young Western and East Asian subjects were tested using fMRI and showed equal presence in both areas of the brain, but when older Western and East Asian subjects were tested for object preference, the East Asian subjects showed significantly less object processing activity in the lateral occipital region (object preference).

What does this mean? Let me start with what we could interpret as an aging effect. Since the young East Asian subjects activated an area of the brain that the older ones did not, the most obvious conclusion is that, because they don't use the object-processing part of the brain as much as Westerners do, it deteriorates with age. And now I'll give you the good news. Since the elderly Asian subjects were told to watch the pictures without receiving any instructions, they used their culturally preferred parahippocampal area (background preference). But . . . when they repeated the test after being given instructions to pay attention to objects rather than backgrounds, they reactivated their lateral occipital area (object preference) without any problems. Thus, rather than cerebral deterioration, it's a culturally biased brain process!

Now that you know the hippocampus is responsible for remembering contextual relationships, I'll tell you about another interesting study. London is not a logically planned city, and the streets have names rather than numbers. So how do London taxi drivers cope? Because they need to memorize complicated contextual references, their hippocampus enlarges to accommodate their challenge. I took a taxi a few months ago in Montevideo, a charming city with winding streets that also are named rather than numbered. I told the driver he probably had a large hippocampus as a result of his line of work. He very happily decided he was going to tell his wife he had a big hippocampus.

My colleague and friend from Harvard, Dr. Ellen Langer, has spent most of her professional career investigating how social context affects aging. In the 1970s, she and her students conducted a study in which a control group of elderly men were told they would attend a retreat where they would spend a week reminiscing about the past. By contrast, the experimental group would spend a week surrounded by paraphernalia from twenty years earlier, listening to radio shows and discussing news from the period. The experimental group was not allowed to bring up any event that happened after 1959, and they were to refer to themselves, their families, and their careers as if they were living before that time. Langer was trying to bring the experimental group into an *as if* context so their thoughts could trigger body signals from their younger days that were dormant in their memories. At the end of the study, the experimental group showed significant improvement in their hearing, eyesight, memory, dexterity, appetite, and other behaviors that supposedly deteriorate with age. Additionally, the experimental group walked away without the aid of canes and carried their own suitcases without the help of family who had assisted them before the study. Interestingly, the reminiscing control group did not achieve the improvements of the experimental one.

Recently, Langer and I discussed her study, and she noted that there had been no mentoring to prevent the mindbody gains the experimental group had made from reverting to age-related *cultural portals*. I consider Ellen one of the most creative researchers in social psychology and, I am pleased to tell you, she now has a center where they teach evidence-based methods to reverse aging and sustain the therapeutic gains. In later chapters I'll extensively discuss why *embodying* beliefs is necessary to affect biological processes. Rather than mind over matter, embodying is the role our body plays in shaping our mind within a cultural context. But it's important to note that the role is reciprocal and culturally influenced.

CULTURAL PSYCHONEUROIMMUNOLOGY

I argue that cultural context is the missing link in PNI research. Instead of continuing to lengthen the name of the interdiscipline each time other biological systems are found to be involved in mindbody communication, and to take PNI out of the lab and into natural cultural settings, I am introducing a new model I call *cultural psychoneuroimmunology*. Although experiments with rats—a substantial area of PNI research—can contribute to our knowledge of how the immune, nervous, and endocrine systems communicate, they are limited to biological data that cannot include psychology, because rats are not human. In other words, cultural beliefs, free will, inspiration, mourning, freedom, honor, admiration, shame, and awareness of our own mortality are important factors that affect human health and longevity—attributes missing in rats!

I am well aware of the argument that rat research allows us to explore biology in ways that would be unethical if human subjects were used, and that we can benefit from some discoveries without sacrificing human life, but my concern is that there is too much focus on rat physiology and next to none on how culture affects the biological systems of human beings. Moreover, PNI research is almost exclusively concerned with the effects of stress and inflammation, and not the *causes of health.*

What do I mean by causes of health? A major limitation in PNI research is the implicit assumption that to achieve health, we have to find how stress harms us so we can learn to cope with, reduce, or eliminate it. This is a legacy from reductionist medicine that defines health as the absence of illness. Throughout this book, I argue that most illnesses are *culturally learned* while the causes of health are *inherited.* With few exceptions, we are born with a body that relentlessly attempts to express our inherited causes of health and a mind that is culturally trained to enhance or limit our potential for sustainable wellness, which is much more than the absence of illness. But I want to be clear that what we inherit are the causes of health, and not health itself. This means *we are born with the potential to both express the constituents of health and to trigger our propensity for illness.*

While I commend the dedication and goodwill of my colleagues who work with rats and humans in order to understand stress, we need to find a balance between exploring what breaks us and what makes us whole. I am also well aware that the discoveries of infectious diseases, vaccines, pharmaceuticals, diagnostics, and many other brilliant contributions of modern science were possible mostly because of research with nonhuman subjects. Hence, rather than replace conventional PNI with cultural psychoneuroimmunology (CPNI), I intend to expand its range of research interests.

A New View of the Immune System

In my opinion, the current model of the immune system is insufficient to explain the complexity of what keeps us healthy. Its proponents maintain that the immune system's purpose is to protect us against foreign bodies in a scenario of constant battle against disease. That sounds reasonable until we ask the following questions: (a) Why does it repair tissue as much as protect us from pathogens? (b) Why does it not reject "foreign bodies" like food, fluids, and medications? (c) Why is it enhanced by positive emotions that have nothing to do with fighting pathogens? (d) Why does it respond selectively to cultural beliefs? And (e), why does it respond based on contextual conditions rather than danger signals?

I'll give you conceptual arguments to keep the technical side light, but if you want more scientific evidence for the model of immune functioning I am proposing, go to the bibliography at the end of this book as well as my published articles on the subject.

Let's examine some historical background to see how the psychological makeup of the scientist who discovered the function of the immune system influenced his interpretation of what he found. Elie Metchnikoff is considered the father of immunology because of his discovery of *phagocytosis*, a cellular response to foreign bodies. Before his finding in 1882, it was thought that white blood cells spread disease rather than fight it. Metchnikoff showed that phagocytes (immune cells) engulfed and destroyed pathogens. As with most significant discoveries, he was first ridiculed for daring to question the wisdom of "established science," and later vindicated with a Nobel Prize in 1908. Metchnikoff was a contemporary of Nietzsche, the great German existential philosopher who proposed that what doesn't kill us makes us stronger. Born a year apart, both brilliant men suffered from severe depression, and attempted suicide several times. My point in mentioning this is that our theories are colored by our cultural history, and immunology is no exception. While Nietzsche concluded that religion is a crutch to diminish our fear of mortality, Metchnikoff offered a model of an immune system that is in constant battle to protect us from a dangerous world. This concept of bellicose functioning continues to limit our understanding of immunology.

The Exalted Emotions

I define the exalted emotions as affects with a foundation in love. They include compassion, empathy, admiration, generosity, gratitude, magnanimity, and any other emotion that expresses our human dignity. But we need a new perspective to understand what the conventional model of the immune system is unable to explain convincingly. I propose that more than protecting us against pathogens, it confirms the operational consciousness we live. Moreover, it makes decisions based on contextual relevance, and not exclusively on differentiating self from nonself. The clonal selection theory, proposed in the late 1950s by Australian immunologist Sir Frank Macfarlane Burnet is the widely accepted model of how the immune system responds to infection. He hypothesized that immunological memory takes place when an immune cell clones two types of cells; one clone acts immediately to fight infection, and the other remains in the system longer to provide immunity against future attacks from the same pathogen—destroy and memorize the intruder. Burnet also proposed that the immune system attacks any foreign body that it identifies as nonself and bypasses everything else—self-identity by default.

But Burnet did not explain why the immune system appears to have a mind of its own when it violates the rules of engagement he proposes in his theory. I believe a battle mindset is what maintains the blind spot. Humanist psychologist Abraham Maslow warned us about the limitations of tunnel visioning: if you only have a hammer, you tend to see every problem as a nail.

David McClelland was one of the first to study how compassion affects the immune system. He showed subjects a fifteen-minute video of Mother Teresa caring for orphans in Calcutta, and found that immunoglobulin type A (IgA) in the saliva increased significantly and remained high for several hours. IgA is an antibody, secreted by B cells, that fights upper respiratory infections like the common cold. Interestingly, the IgAs remained high only in subjects who were also asked to think about their own acts of kindness.

Several studies that replicated McClelland's show consistent increases in IgA as well as other immune-protecting cells they measured. Many other studies confirm that the immune system responds to positive emotions in a way that cannot be explained using the conventional model. In other words, if IgAs are antibodies that are released to fight pathogens, why do they respond when we experience compassion? In my biocognitive model of the immune system, I suggest that exalted emotions trigger immune enhancement to corroborate the operative consciousness of humane connection we experience, rather than to fight viruses.

Thus, the immune system *confirms* the mindbody existence we choose to express. Other studies also verify that when we embody memories from our own experiences, our immune and other systems respond accordingly. In other words, the positive IgA response from watching Mother Teresa's video was prolonged when subjects recalled their own acts of compassion because it consolidated their experience.

Oxytocin is a hormone and neurotransmitter produced mainly in the pituitary gland. It has gained popularity as a prescription drug because of its association with bonding, monogamy, and love. This does not mean, however, that those behaviors are *caused by* oxytocin—though that's the dream of some pharmaceutical companies that conclude that, because a chemical is found in a behavior, it's the cause of it, and consequently they can synthesize it and make fortunes selling it as the latest wonder drug. Fortunately, though, that's not how it works. Rather than magic pills, the coauthorship of your thoughts, emotions, and biology is what determines the joy or misery in your life. You are the architect and pharmacist of your own destiny. For example, your body creates endorphins, a peptide more powerful than heroin or any other narcotic, and although they are readily produced through exercise and contemplative methods, some choose to ruin their lives with dangerous synthesized drugs—the external quick fix for whatever ails you. As you continue reading this book, I will frequently assure you that I am not against medications or the pharmaceutical companies that produce them. Nor am I against financial benefits accruing from worthy contributions to science. My argument is against those who profit from the misery of others by selling chemicals that can be accessed from within.

Let's return to oxytocin and explore its legitimate value. Its role in human emotions is made more relevant than its discovery by observing bonding behavior in animals. Oxytocin is released during breast-feeding and lovemaking, and when we feel admiration, trust, optimism, monogamous love, and many more bonding experiences. But let's also look at what goes on in the underlying biological terrain. Oxytocin is anti-inflammatory, helps immune cells fight bacteria, improves digestion, inhibits growth of malignant cells, increases efficiency of endocrine response to infection, helps repair heart tissue, and much more.

Conversely, oxytocin is low or absent in post-traumatic stress disorder, autism, childhood trauma, betrayal, and other conditions and behaviors that disrupt social bonding.

But again, we need to question how these PNI benefits fit into the immunology model whose main purpose is to fight pathogens and identify what is foreign to the body. I suggest that the model does not jibe because it lacks two important components: contextual relevance and rules for non-battle conditions. Viewing the immune system as protector of self and destroyer of nonself precludes exploring possibilities outside these rigid boundaries. This is one of the reasons why conventional PNI is almost exclusively concerned with what the immune system fights instead of what we love. The *confirming* model of immune function I propose can cogently explain why our biology responds differently when we love than when we fear. It's more about corroborating our humanity than survival of our species.

The HIV viruses (there at least two types) specifically infect CD4 T cells. These T helper cells, as they're called, orchestrate complex immune defenses. When the virus destroys a significant number of T helper cells, it leaves the patient susceptible to infection and disease. Thus, AIDS (acquired immune deficiency syndrome) begins when the immune system can no longer fight opportunistic infections and tumors. Rather than the virus, the *acquired* immune insufficiency is what promotes illnesses that eventually kill the patient.

Working with HIV-positive patients, George Solomon discovered that assertiveness positively affects T helper cell levels. The more assertive (able to set reasonable emotional limits) patients had higher levels of T cells in their blood. By the way, I argue that assertiveness is one of the causes of health. Other studies have replicated Solomon's findings and found that forgiveness also increases immune function of HIV-positive patients. In other words, HIV-positive patients who genuinely forgive the person who infected them live longer than those who hold on to their grudges. (I dedicate all of chapter 8 to teaching you how to successfully forgive because forgiveness is so widely misunderstood and is vital to healing. In fact, I am convinced that forgiveness is one of the most important causes of health.)

Candice Pert, a microbiologist who discovered endorphin receptors, also found that the vasoactive intestinal peptide (VIP) protects T helper cells by blocking the HIV virus. She speculated the VIP may be triggered by love and other bonding behaviors similar to what stimulates oxytocin. Although there is next to no research with human subjects on the psychoneuroimmunology of VIP, we know the peptide facilitates oxytocin release; both are secreted from the pituitary gland and are involved in the regulation of serotonin, a neurotransmitter considered one of the causes of clinical depression when its levels drop rapidly. VIP is also produced in the hypothalamus, and if you decide to look deeper into psychoneuroimmunology research, you will find that both stress and antistress hormones, peptides, and neurotransmitters are found in the three glands that make up the HPA axis. This means that stress is interpreted based on context and cultural history rather than on conditions existing outside of yourself.

Let's build on the example I used in the last chapter of encountering a lion. If you are in a conference room listening to a lecture on global warming, and suddenly a lion steps into the room, you and most of the audience will experience a stress response. Is the lion a stressor? It depends on context and cultural history. If you were instead attending a lecture to learn lion taming, you would most likely welcome the lion. And if the same lion were to step up to a group of Masai (East African tribe) adolescents, they would see the lion as an opportunity for them to protect their cattle and show courage. Although killing a lion as a rite of passage is a myth, Masai adolescents learn early to defend their herds from lions and other predatory animals. Portuguese slave traders bypassed the fearless Masai warriors because they realized it was not good business to mess with them. Thus, true to the two Chinese characters that signify stress, the lion is both danger and opportunity.

The Primitive Emotions

What I call *primitive emotions* are founded in dysfunctional fear, and are on the side opposite that of the exalted. Fear is a physiological response that is necessary to signal danger and warn us to proceed with caution, but other than those adaptive functions, it does not serve us well because it alienates us from love. If we embrace fear beyond its adaptive purpose, it grows into anger, hatred, jealousy, resentment, envy, greed, shame, and other primitive emotions that disconnect us from the best we have to offer.

You already know that the exalted emotions enhance immune function, and how they fit into the biocognitive model. Now I want to show you how the primitive emotions affect your health. The immune system is a bioinformation field of glands and lymphatic pathways that responds to internal and external contextual challenges. My proposal that the immune system has a moral code, however, is the most important concept in this chapter, so I will elaborate my argument as clearly as I am able, and hope you will join me with an open mind.

THE MORAL IMMUNE SYSTEM

When I speak of morality, I am not referring to self-righteous rules invoked by those who are intolerant of others who don't meet their rigid standards of conduct. Instead, I am describing a moral code that differentiates between the exalted and primitive emotions. More specifically, I propose that the immune system thrives when we experience bonding emotions, and declines when we live in fear. This can happen only if it can discern the difference using a moral code that favors love over fear and compassion over hatred.

The moral immune system is enhanced when we present it with emotions founded in love that confirm that we are expressing our nobleness. But if we choose a life of fear-based emotions, it can also confirm the worst in us. Either way, rather than judging or protecting us, it responds to the path we choose for our journey.

How can glands and lymphatic nodes have morals? If you reduce them to their parts, they're mere tissues that communicate biochemically—no morality there. And that is the reductionists' argument, using reasoning tools borrowed from Newtonian mechanics. But I don't want to give you esoteric explanations from the other extreme either, such as subtle energy communication, quantum wisdom, human vibrations, and other concepts that may sound aesthetically pleasing but lack the practical answers I want you to have. In other words, the reductionist argument is too narrow, and the universal one is too wide. Both leave you wondering what to do with their explanations.

Biocognitive science takes the middle way to converge the best from each side and formulate useful answers. To illustrate, animals have more *epigenetic communication* than humans because they don't have language to convey danger. We lost most of our capacity to communicate biologically when we invented language. Rats, for example, don't have the advantage of being able to tell their offspring that some foods are poisonous.

Before I proceed with more examples, I'll briefly explain epigenetics from the technical and practical sides. Epigenetics is "the study of heritable changes in gene activity that are *not* caused by changes in the DNA sequence." This means that vital information *learned* by one generation is genetically transferred to the next. Before epigenetics was discovered, it was thought that genes could not learn because the DNA codes that express them do not provide that option. In other words, DNA is the blueprint that determines gene expression, but epigenetics and other mindbody research is showing that the expression is affected by contextual conditions; Mother Nature sets rules to be questioned, not to be blindly obeyed.

One of several studies illustrates how rats communicate epigenetically. After allowing two rats to groom each other (establish bonding), the experimenters separated them and gave one of the rats poisoned food, enough to make it sick without killing it. After the two rats groomed each other again, when the healthy rat was offered food with the same poison, it refused to eat it. More remarkably, the offspring of both rats were offered the poisoned food not long after they were born, and they refused it as well (epigenetic transfer of vital information).

What we lost in epigenetic capabilities, we gained in language that allows us to communicate our fear and joy. We advanced from survival biology to biocognitive meaning. When a parent tells a child something is dangerous, the symbol representing danger is assimilated biosymbolically. The amygdala (fear-registry gland) codes the information as a biological signal of danger, while other parts of the brain archive the linguistic characteristics of the word (sound and meaning). Thus, nonhuman species store events from their senses, and we from the sensations and emotions signaled by our language. For instance, a cultural editor (mother, teacher, or chef) tells you *galerina* mushrooms are deadly poisonous, look like umbrellas with rusty-brown, circular caps, and usually grow on rotting wood. What happens with all this information? (a) You hear the warning with undivided attention because it comes from an authority figure who mentions the words *deadly* and *poisonous;* (b) your brain creates a semantic space with the name, color, form, sound, and context of the danger; (c) the semantic space incorporates the sensations and emotions elicited by the warning; and (d) the *cluster* of semantics, emotions, and sensations is stored as a biosymbol in archives of memories with similar characteristics of danger.

The biosymbol is archived like *fractals* in different parts of the brain, without breaking its connections, like unwinding a bundle of strings without cutting them. Each component is stored according to its individual characteristics: sound in the temporal lobe, words in the left hemisphere, spatial relations in the right hemisphere, danger sensations in the amygdalae, context in the hippocampus, visual imagery in the occipital cortex, and abstracted meaning in the frontal lobe. These locations are not important to remember unless you're interested in neuropsychology, but I want you to understand that the brain does not function isolated from the immune, endocrine, nervous, and other systems, because the mind is more than the brain. The apparently simple warning about poisonous mushrooms enters a bioinformational field in which language and biology coauthor meaning from head to toes.

Let's see what happens with our immune system when a word with cultural weight enters our bioinformational field. Several studies in PNI indicate that shame causes inflammation! Sally Dickerson and Margaret Kemeny asked subjects to write for fifteen minutes about instances when they felt shamed. The experimenters measured, in the subjects' saliva, pre- and post- levels of a molecule called *tumor necrosis factor* (TNF). Tumor necrosis factor, a reliable indicator of inflammation, is usually triggered by infection and other immunological damage. The post- measurements of the experimental group showed significant increases in TNF levels after fifteen minutes of recalling shameful memories. How is that possible? How can the word *shame* cause an immune system response akin to infection? Conventional PNI does not explain how a word creates biology, but I believe the biosymbolic prepping I am giving you in this chapter will yield credible answers.

I know you're getting the picture, but now I'll provide more examples of cultural PNI to give you a deeper understanding of the biocognitive model of immunology. In Peru and other South American countries, *bochorno* is the word used for the hot flashes of menopause. In Spanish, *bochorno* means "shame." And by now, you know that shame causes inflammation. In contrast, Japanese women use the word *konenki*, meaning "turn or change of life," and in Chinese medicine, menopause is diagnosed as the *second spring*. South American women who experience their hot flashes as shame have significantly more inflammatory problems, painful symptoms, hormone replacement therapy, and diminished sense of beauty than Japanese and Chinese women, who welcome menopause as a natural transition to the second spring of their lives. I argue that, in general, our biology adjusts to our cultural beliefs; and in particular, our immune system confirms the operative consciousness with which we choose to view our world. I will have more to say throughout the book about operative consciousness, but for now think of it as the goggles you use to see and interpret what goes on in your life.

The Contextual Immune System

I also propose in the biocognitive model that the immune system makes decisions based on context, not by differentiating self from nonself. The conventional model appears reasonable because it correctly shows, in elegant detail, how antibodies fight pathogens and remember the pathogens' characteristics to prepare for future intrusions—so far, no argument. The problem surfaces when the rules of engagement do not hold—for instance, when antibodies and other defense mechanisms do not attack nonself entities, do not detect danger, do not respond to injured tissue, and display many other conditions that indicate something other than rigid rules of attack are guiding the system. The conventional model confuses cause and effect. In other words, nonself recognition is the cause it attributes to the attack response rather than the context in which the recognition takes place.

But if we consider context as the cause for action, it explains why: (a) benign bacteria are not attacked, (b) bacteria that cause duodenal ulcers (H. pylori) are not confronted until they reach certain levels, (c) some people with the rheumatoid factor (RF) do not develop rheumatoid arthritis, (d) some tumors are not detected, (e) cultural names given to biological processes (such as menopause) determine immune response, (f) righteous anger is good for the immune system, and (g) words from physicians and shamans can heal or kill in their respective contexts of power. I could go on to fill a book, but you get the point.

Let's look at a few compelling examples that show how context determines action. You know that IgAs are antibodies that destroy viruses, but you may not know how their function changes based on contextual relevance. Although food, fluids, and medications are "foreign bodies," we ingest them without objection from our immune system. How is that possible? Because, since these conditions have nutritional and healing contextual relevance, the immune system does not fight them. But I'll be more specific with how IgAs work contextually when we eat, drink, and take medication.

Here are the contextual rules that allow us to absorb these items: (a) the ingestion has to be oral; (b) to prevent pathogens, it must *not* include proliferating organisms; and (c) it must be wrapped with IgAs. Thus, IgAs play an important role in digestion because in that context, they go from fighting pathogens to protecting food and medication. When the food arrives at the small intestine (where most of the digestion takes place), it's surveyed by Peyer's patches (lymphatic tissue) to detect any pathogens in the food—like a checkpoint. If it meets the criteria, the food, fluid, or medication is allowed to proceed. Interestingly, the IgAs wrapped in the food function as immune suppressors rather than antibodies. In other words, they tell the immune system not to attack because the context is different.

But . . . if while you're digesting dinner at a fine restaurant, the chef approaches your table with fear in her eyes and tells you the food is poisoned, all bets are off, and you'll soon be running to the nearest bathroom to expel the food from one end or the other. Again, words from authorities (cultural editors) impact biology with a placebo or nocebo effect: I shall heal, or I shall harm.

There's extensive literature documenting incidents of people who have died because of misdiagnosis of terminal illness, a voodoo curse, a life-expectancy chart, autosuggestion, and many other nocebo effects. Conversely, some people who believe in the power of a professional, a medication, or prayer to make tumors disappear live significantly longer than prognosticated and heal from "incurable" illness.

❖ ❖ ❖

I am glad you stuck with me through a complex chapter that requires shifting your mindset, challenging mechanistic science, and taking off those goggles that limit your potential for living a long and healthy life. The immune system has morals, but the good news is that you coauthor the rules of engagement. Some you learn from your culture, and others you assimilate from your own experiences, but now you can proceed, armed with scientific evidence, to respectfully challenge the cultural editors who limit your joy.

Guardians of the Heart

This chapter is about the kinds of deeply loving relationships we experience when we become *guardians of the heart*.

I see relationships as opportunities to heal archetypal wounds. They are also opportunities to coauthor belonging without ownership and love without fear. Guardianship in relationships celebrates the union of two individuals who commit to a *covenant of safety* that promotes mutual emotional healing and resolves the fear of being wounded again. But to be a guardian of the heart is about much more than healing wounds. The covenant of safety we create is a foundation we establish so we may communicate the language of love without the obstruction of archetypal wounds. If you commit to protecting your partner's heart, and you trust your partner to protect yours, you achieve the two objectives of the covenant of safety: trust and dignity. It's an indirect way to learn worthiness, commitment, and faith, all through the power of love.

To be guardians of the heart differs from what I call *ledger relationships* in which partners focus on keeping score: giving while expecting to receive, and taking while expecting to give back. Although this type of exchange may seem reasonable, when you look deeper, you see transactions of *giving* and *taking* with hidden agendas rather than *offering* and *receiving* for the pure joy of experiencing the exchange. When we offer, we endow without expecting anything back; and when we receive, we accept without having to give anything back. The real gifts are the gratitude we experience when we receive, and the generosity we feel when we offer.

RESOLVING YOUR FEAR OF
BEING WOUNDED AGAIN

In chapter 2, you learned how the three archetypal wounds—abandonment, shame, and betrayal—create helplessness, and how their respective healing fields of commitment, honor, and loyalty empower. Abandonment disempowers because it breaks a pledge, shame disempowers because it degrades, and betrayal disempowers because it severs devotion. Healing from these wounds is about you, not about fixing the person who wounded you. And as you know by now, healing is not a thought process. It is an embodiment of the felt meaning in the corresponding healing field. Relationships offer an opportunity to bring healthy closure to unresolved wounds—a scenario to work through the unworthiness you learned from your cultural editors. If you enter relationships without committing to coauthoring personal development, you will let your painful history confuse the challenges of your present with the wounding ghosts from your past. When you overreact emotionally, it's usually a signal that your response comes from your history of wounds; for example, if your partner is fifteen minutes late for dinner, you react with such intensity that you might just as well have been abandoned on a deserted island.

Guardians of the heart consciousness teaches you to coauthor worthiness with a partner who is willing to see your painful, unfinished business as an opportunity to recontextualize your fear of being wounded again, a willingness you extend to your partner as well. But fear of opening your heart cannot be resolved by a guarantee that you are not going to be wounded again. Instead, resolution comes while you are coauthoring healing fields of commitment, honor, and loyalty, endorsing a covenant of safety that allows both of you to work through your mistakes, and find wisdom in your imperfection.

These lofty goals can only be reached if you decide to be worthy rather than right. The satisfaction of besting your partner will never exceed the joy of knowing you took the honorable road instead.

HORIZONTAL AND VERTICAL LOVE

Horizontal love remains superficial. *Vertical love* goes deep.

Horizontal lovers seek quantity, are emotionally shallow, and view their most recent "soul mate" as a temporary experience of intensity, to be traded in for another one when the partner begins to demand emotional substance. Horizontal lovers are committed to noncommitment. They have many acquaintances and few friends. Their archetypal wounds run deep, and when they surface, these lovers usually project them on to others rather than take ownership. Although horizontal lovers are very likable and fun to be around, and they appear to take an interest in their relationships, all their positive attributes vanish when they are asked to keep the commitments they have made to share their future.

Guardians of the heart are all about vertical love. Vertical lovers seek quality and emotional depth; they take soul mates for better or for worse, until death. This does not mean they remain in abusive or toxic relationships—this is *co*authorship, not a one-way street. Vertical lovers never cease to find novelty in their partners. You can find vertical love in partners who have spent a lifetime together and still laugh at each other's jokes, and continue to express admiration for the beauty they see in their relationship. They will never use a social opportunity to ridicule one another. Vertical lovers sustain passion when the body grows old, maintain faith in workable outcomes during the darkest moments, and mourn their end with gratitude and resolve.

What I am describing is not a fairy tale; guardians of the heart are found everywhere. I have witnessed the positive attributes I am inviting you to learn in this chapter in many long-lasting, healthy relationships I have known and studied worldwide. I say *healthy* relationships because I see little value in long-term relationships from hell. A shared history is not a sufficient foundation for vertical love.

THE THREE STAGES OF VERTICAL LOVE

Many divorces are avoidable, and most relationships do not have to inevitably become a struggle to be understood. Most problematic relationships lack the *tools of love* required to overcome challenges; they do not lack love itself. Love is always necessary, but it is not sufficient to make relationships work. Yet it's easier to understand that pilots require navigational instruments to fly safely through storms than it is to recognize that intimate relationships are learned interactions with cultural rules. We know pilots require special training, but we may not know that we communicate in our relationships using an intimate language of love we learned from our cultural editors. If we were taught to fear love, we are unprepared to embrace it. Pilots and lovers both require navigational charts to overcome their respective storms.

I propose there are three stages involved in developing competence in the intimate language of love: *attraction, engagement,* and *embracement.* To attract simply requires triggering inquisitive interest. Engaging goes further and demands aesthetic compatibility. And embracing transcends the personal horizons of each participant so they may merge the best histories they have assimilated from the collective wisdom of their respective cultures. When we skip one stage or lack competence in one before progressing to another, we arrive without the tools to overcome the challenges that are unique to that stage; in other words, each stage has its own characteristic storms as well as tools we can use to navigate through them.

Attraction

In this initial stage, we are drawn by curiosity about the attributes and qualities we find in the other person. This can take the form of physical attraction, intellectual admiration, emotional compatibility, mystery, or something we lack or find desirable in the other person. We show our best behavior to attract this person, and we enter a domain of friendship. The attraction stage requires gradual emotional and intellectual contribution to building a friendship, and we create our first storm in this stage when we conclude that we should be lovers because we are good friends. We are most vulnerable to premature intimacy of this kind when we enter the relationship with loneliness.

Horizontal lovers seldom progress to the next two stages. Patience and prudence are the two navigational tools we must put to use to avoid the storms that brew from impulsiveness. The lesson is clear: attraction is an invitation to engage rather than engagement itself.

Engagement

We enter this stage after we have established a friendship with mutual trust. While the first stage was about determining mutual attraction, in the engagement stage, we go beyond what we like about each other to explore together what we like about the world. Here we look for compatibility concerning external aesthetics: music, politics, religion, socioeconomics, ethics, social rules, prejudices, and other contextual conditions that shape our world.

Compatibility, though, is not the same as agreement. We can have different views on any of the aesthetic factors of this stage as long as we also have tolerance for our differences. Here we want to develop the grace to agree to disagree, without bruising our egos. The most common storm in this stage is triggered when we look for an exact replica of our worldview rather than aesthetic diversity. *Mature tolerance* is the most potent tool we can use to navigate smoothly in the engagement stage. I want to be clear, however, that tolerance does not mean submissiveness or suppressing our own aesthetics. *Mature tolerance means honoring our partner's aesthetics without shaming our own.* Later I'll have more to say about the danger of compromising your values.

Embracement

After we explore our personal attractions and aesthetic compatibilities with our friend and future partner, we can enter the embracement stage. Here we embrace a new subculture based on the best of our respective histories. We include our tribal rituals of honor, commitment, and loyalty; exclude the wounding patterns we learned from our cultural editors; and begin to live a fusion of what is best in our respective cultures. As we embrace the best and discard the worst of our patterns for dealing with life, we also select the coauthors we want to include and those we want to release.

Discarding toxic coauthors involves both literal and figurative action. Some toxic authors live in our world, and others live in our minds. Both types of coauthors have to go if you want to give embracement a fair chance. (Of course, you may wish to maintain some ties with toxic family members, and if you do so, I suggest you limit the time you spend with them.)

The storms in this stage strike when you relentlessly impose your cultural beliefs on your partner. Cultural diversity is the most effective tool for navigating the storm of that type of imposition. Embracement consciousness allows you to expand your cultural beliefs without having to endure punishment from your old coauthors of unworthiness.

If you are wondering at which of the three stages you should begin to work on healing your archetypal wounds, I congratulate you on your timing—you may uncover and work with a wound at any of the three stages. Although the stages are sequential, they don't have to be experienced mechanically. Remember, all fields are contained by fluid horizons that allow you to transition smoothly from field to field. Since these three stages are interwoven mindbody fields, you can return to areas that require more work without necessarily regressing back to those stages. If you are in the second or third stage, the advantage of returning to earlier stages for additional refinement is that you will be moved by love and inspired by the infinite verticality of your relationship. Your relationship will never weaken if you navigate old storms with new (appropriate) tools.

ENTERING YOUR HEALING FIELDS
DURING TURBULENT TIMES

As you continue to read this book, you will find that I present concepts and tools based on complex circumstances and scenarios that are far from ideal. In fact, biocognitive theory and practice partly evolved from the trenches where life is rough, the future seems dim, and the coauthors of unworthiness are plentiful. But it does not follow that you can only learn from misery. Instead, your journey here requires confronting your fears, disillusionments, and learned helplessness with tools that harness hope—tools based on scientific evidence rather than wishful thinking. I bring you good news in the form of methods that require a commitment to finding your joy, not quick fixes.

By the way, if you are not in a romantic relationship at the moment, you are not excluded from practicing guardianship of the heart. Celibate clergy and committed singles alike can apply the same principles.

Why does it work for all? Because guardianship is about the relationship you create with yourself and extend to your partner, if you choose to have a partner. In the case of celibate clergy, their personal relationship is extended to God. Atheists can extend it to Nature or anything they consider worthy beyond the self, and singles can extend it to how they treat themselves.

Now let's look at how you can enter the healing fields during turbulent times in relationship with yourself and with partners. Effective tools actually work best under difficult conditions because they are designed to handle worst-case scenarios. It's easy to make almost anything work when things are going well, but when you're confronted with challenges that feel overwhelming, it's easy to forget your newly learned alternatives and regress to the dysfunctional patterns you know so well—and that lead to failure. My point here is that guardians of the heart consciousness enhances your relationship with yourself and others when things are going well, when turbulence emerges, and even when you forget to use the tools, because it is more than a set of techniques.

Let's continue to conceptually explore navigating healing fields before you dive into practical applications at the end of the chapter.

Turbulence in a relationship is a two-way street. It is created when you are unwilling to engage your partner's healing field, or when your partner is unwilling to engage yours. For example, let's say that you realize you just shamed your partner by something you said at a party. Having committed to being a guardian of the heart and recognizing your mistake, you faithfully enter the field of honor to correct it, but find that your partner is unwilling to accept your offer. What can you do? First, you can recognize that an offer of honor does not lose its healing power when the person you have wounded refuses it. It is intrinsically honorable, independent of the response you get. Remember, you are trying to heal *your* wounding behavior, not attempting to heal your partner. You behave honorably to elevate your conduct, not to be rewarded with understanding and appreciation. Also, you are inviting your partner to enter the healing field of honor with you, and consequently, it is your partner's responsibility to accept or reject your offer.

Here is a possible narrative of what could happen:

YOU "I am sorry I joked about your weight. What can I do to
show you my love?"

YOUR PARTNER "There's not a damn thing you can do! Just leave
me alone."

YOU "I understand. Whenever you're ready to accept my apology,
let me know."

Your partner feels hurt and understandably does not want instant resolution; it takes time to recuperate from an emotional hit. Meanwhile, you avoid inflicting further wounding and taking responsibility for fixing your partner.

Eventually, if your partner does not use the situation to manipulate you by playing the victim, he or she will accept your honorable offer of apology. Healing fields are entered into without hidden agendas.

Being mindful of giving your partner time to recover from an insult such as this can also help you recognize your own need to recover when you are insulted. And interestingly, when you give yourself permission to take time to recover, you shorten the time it takes, and you become aware of any ways in which you are misusing that time to manipulate by playing the victim.

THE TRAPS OF VICTIMHOOD

If you are raped or otherwise physically abused, you are victimized. However, if you use this or any other painful circumstance to control and manipulate others, you enter victimhood. When you are victimized, you need understanding and compassion. By contrast, when you are in victimhood, you demand pity. Compassion heals because it is a legitimate offer of love. Demand for pity feeds a kind of manipulative helplessness because it is disingenuous. If you feel anger toward someone who has suffered abuse, when you think you should feel compassion, it is most likely because you are being manipulated with victimhood. Even if this is happening, though, be mindful not to become callous because you're afraid to open your heart. It may be that you are expressing anger when compassion is more appropriate because you are unwilling to acknowledge your partner's legitimate pain.

One morning, when I was making rounds at a psychiatric hospital, I experienced a striking example of victimhood. A patient I was going to see had been exempted—with staff's blessings—from attending group therapy and other required activities. Anytime staff referred to this patient, they expressed pity for the poor man's plight. When I walked into the patient's room to interview him, the first thing I saw on his dresser was a photo of a baby in a casket. Immediately, I felt overwhelming sorrow for that unfortunate man.

I started the usual mental status exam and eventually broached the most difficult topic. "I noticed the picture on your dresser. Tell me what happened." In the telling, the patient contorted his face oddly, an expression I could not understand at the moment, but one that put me on alert and let me know that I was pitying him rather than feeling compassion. He told me his only son had died suddenly of a rare disease. After a few more questions, and acknowledging his pain, I asked, "When did your son pass away?"

"Ten years ago," he said.

That was my first wake-up call. I asked if he had more children, and he said he had two other children but had not been very close with them because of "his pain." The picture I had of him now turned from that of a bereaved father to a self-centered man who was depriving his living children of his love.

Please understand that I can only imagine the overwhelming pain of losing a child. What I want to illustrate with this story is the manipulation of pain, not the disregarding of it. While in the hospital, this patient was avoiding therapy that could help him, and instead was asking for special meals and other privileges. At home, he was depriving his other children of fatherly love and making his wife the sole breadwinner. But here is the proof of his victimhood: when I told him he had to attend group therapy and other required activities, he asked to be discharged because we could not understand his pain!

RECONTEXTUALIZING BOREDOM
IN YOUR RELATIONSHIP

I want to give boredom special attention in this chapter because it is one of the most frequent reasons I hear for disillusionment, at best, and betrayal, at worst, in failing relationships.

We live in societies that idealize beauty, wit, wealth, sexuality, humor, fame, and other attributes that are continually and aggressively marketed by an array of media. We mere mortals can never live up to the standards of our modern cultural gods. And although we realize intellectually that these "perfect" characters we are bombarded with are nothing more than marketed dreams, we may privately wish we could find someone who comes close to such a fantasized partner. If we share our life with the "mortal" partner we have chosen, hoping the person will approximate the god or goddess we want, it's not difficult to see how boredom can creep in to confirm our disappointment.

Can boredom be avoided? Fortunately, no! Boredom can help us realize that we are creating reruns within our relationships. It can be a signal of our stagnation. Reruns may indicate that we are taking our partner's attributes for granted, or becoming what we disliked about our parents, or comparing apples to oranges in the ways we think about our partner. These are all obvious reasons for boredom that you can find in any self-help book. The mindset shift I propose here is very different. Here we are going to discover the navigational dynamics of vertical love.

Vertical love seeks depth, and we see our partner as a universe filled with endless potential for discovery. What you may not know about navigating vertical love is that what you call "boredom" is actually a *novelty plateau* in your journey of discovery. Independent of how creative you are, you will encounter repetitive patterns in yourself and your partner that can dampen your enthusiasm. Just as markets have periods of contraction after ones of consistent growth, our journey of vertical love has novelty plateaus at which we tire of communication that has lost its initial function. What was initially witty has lost its funny punch line, what was once refreshing has turned stale, and what was exciting has become predictable. Why? Because fields of bioinformation require replenishment, and communication without novelty is a signal they have been depleted. When horizontal lovers get to this point, they leave before breaking through these repetitive loops. Since vertical lovers are in it for the long run, they conclude that boredom is part of the package and decide to endure the reruns. But I offer another option for those who choose to joyfully stay. If you can recontextualize boredom as a novelty plateau, there are ways to replenish spent fields of bioinformation and revitalize your relationship.

Breaking Through Novelty Plateaus

You have learned that boredom is a signal that you are playing reruns and need something new. In chapter 2, you also learned that recontextualizing a concept means changing its felt meaning rather than replacing one word for another. One problem we have in modifying our behavior is that it requires more than replacing semantics; we are more than our language and our thoughts. We are mindbody, sentient beings in cultural contexts.

Now, you may ask, "If you're trying to free me of my boring reruns, why are you repeating such concepts throughout the book?" Like all legitimate questions, this one deserves a cogent response, and the answer is that repetition alone does not cause boredom; the novelty plateau is the culprit.

So what's the difference? When you reach a novelty plateau, you are repeating what you say or do *without expanding the meaning* of what is being repeated. In fact, one of the key methods I am applying to teach you new concepts is a special use of repetition based on how our brain learns best. I call it *biocognitive iteration.* I borrowed the term *iteration* from chaos theory, and in my work, it means repeating a sequence of operations to successively expand the contextual felt meaning of a symbol. So each repetition of a concept you encounter here adds new information to expand and deepen your felt meaning of the concept. For example, a pencil is an instrument usually used to write with. But a pencil could also be a stick you use to stir your coffee. It could be a weapon to stab someone who is trying to kill you. These are some iterations of the meaning of pencil. But on the novelty plateau, a pencil is and will forever be merely a writing instrument.

Some people in relationships break through their boredom naturally, without knowing they are engaging in the dynamics you will learn here. But most of us can benefit from learning what some others practice intuitively. The guidance I offer here can enhance your journey and cut short the personal storms you experience along the way.

Here is a practical example. A few years ago I taught a neuropsychology course to a group of professional interior designers to show them how the brain makes decisions regarding the aesthetics of space. I was teaching them some of the rules they already applied intuitively, despite not knowing *how* their brains went about choosing color, perspective, and transitions from room to room. They intuitively chose greens and blues for bedrooms, yellow hues for kitchens, and wood for libraries. When I asked them to give me reasons for their choices, they would respond, "It feels right" or "It creates harmony."

They were navigating with experience and good taste. But I knew that if I could teach them how the brain makes aesthetic decisions, they could improve their "intuition." And that is exactly what happened. For example, blues and greens go well together because the three primary colors—red, blue, and yellow—determine complementarity. Based on how our brain processes color from the retina to the visual cortex, the best-fit rule for primary and complementary colors is that a primary color goes best with what the remaining two primary colors produce when they mix. Red goes best with green because when you mix the remaining two primary colors, blue and yellow, you get green. Yellow goes best with purple because mixing the two remaining primary colors, red and blue, makes purple, and so on. The interior design students were delighted to learn some of the things I had explained about color: that pregnant women and children prefer hues of purple, for example, but that after the mother gives birth and the child grows up, purple ceases to be a favorite. The new insights I was able to share added novelty to the designers' experience of their field.

To finish my quick lesson on neuropsychology of interior design, you might want to know that yellow hues trigger creativity, blues and greens reduce blood pressure, and wood can symbolize authority and intellectual contemplation, hence its use in courtrooms and home libraries.

Now let's return to our topic, novelty plateaus, to look at how your brain creates and resolves boredom.

It's Monday morning, and you wake up to heavy rain, foreboding lightning, and booming thunderclaps. You say to your partner, "What a lovely day. It inspires me to go outside and dance in the rain." Your partner laughs, enjoying the novelty of your statement, and appreciates the way you lightened what had begun as a moody start to the week. Then, because it was a funny thing to say and your partner was delighted, you repeat it every time it rains (contextual repetition). Before long the brain is on automatic pilot, and what was initially a delightful and unexpected moment you shared becomes boring.

When the brain reaches such a novelty plateau, it's asking for new information. It wants to maintain the levels of exploration and discovery it requires to function well. So, if you recognize boredom as a signal from your brain that it needs new food for thought, you have a choice: you can feed it with discovery or keep starving it with reruns. In the practical applications section later in the chapter, I'll teach you ways to break free of novelty plateaus and celebrate the wisdom that underlies your boredom.

COMPROMISE IS FOR LEDGER RELATIONSHIPS

Some books on relationships teach you how to compromise with your partner. If you like art shows and your partner likes basketball, one week you endure a basketball game, and the following week you drag your partner to an art exhibit.

Does that seem reasonable? It does if you choose to live in a ledger relationship, in which partners think in terms of assets and liabilities. If you take a good, hard, honest look, you may have to admit that when you compromise your personal joy, mutual enjoyment diminishes; you feel guilty for making your partner do what you like to do and resentful when you have to do what you don't like. One of the flaws in a compromise approach is making the assumption that in a relationship, you have to enjoy everything together. Tit for tat may work well for balance sheets, but it's a setup for getting stuck at novelty plateaus in healthy relationships.

Although there are times when common sense dictates an art show one day and a ballgame the next, if compromise is the rule rather than the exception in your relationship, guilt and resentment will become the currency you exchange on the ledger.

Another common suggestion is the win-win alternative, and that can be nice because you can choose something both partners enjoy. But if this becomes your go-to choice, you can enjoy only what you like to do together, and consequently you will neglect your personal preferences in order to please your partner. You will give up your unique *joy finger-print*—the things that especially excite you as an individual and make you come alive—and instead your relationship will become your identity. Well, is that so bad? Yes it is, if you want joy in your relationship without having to compromise your individual passion.

When I was in private practice, the most frequent complaint I heard in marital conflicts was "I can't do some things I love anymore because my partner hates them." See how the win-win solution leaves no room for each individual's joy fingerprint?

The best solution is to fold personal life into your interpersonal relationship. The goodwill you build when you leave your partner free to enjoy something in your absence will greatly enhance what you choose to enjoy together. In the next section, I will address potential problems when "my joy in your absence" is misused.

BELONGINGNESS WITHOUT OWNERSHIP

I respect anthropological differences, so in this discussion I will tailor my suggestions to people whose cultural belief is that relationships do not equal ownership, as well as to those who wish to break from any tribal rules that oppress them when they seek equity in relationships. If you are still with me—believing that the partners in a relationship do not own each other—let's continue your lessons in biocognition.

Slavery was outlawed worldwide many years ago, yet many people continue to implicitly believe that love equals ownership. When you hear them say "my woman" or "my man," they mean it literally—this person belongs to me. Interestingly, when you say those same words to express *belongingness* rather than ownership, the felt meaning changes from oppression to sensuality.

Since ownership in relationships is based on fear, any attempt to express your joy fingerprint in such cases can trigger one or more archetypal wounds; if you want to enjoy something by yourself, it must be because you want to abandon, shame, or betray your partner. Although trust is an antidote to ownership in relationships, another component feeds fear in relationships: a cultural belief that you have to be everything for your partner. If joy is missing in your partner's life, only you can provide it. Or it can only happen in your presence. To be a good partner in a relationship, you must monopolize the other person's joy.

This need to monopolize increases if your partner abuses the freedom you offer; for example, flirting with others when you're not around. I cannot emphasize enough that everything I teach in this chapter can only work if you and your partner commit to guarding each other's hearts. The covenant of safety you agree to uphold is fundamental to exploring belongingness without ownership. You belong together by choice, relinquish your monopoly of the other's joy, and draw on creativity and love to dignify your differences. Your felt meaning transitions from belonging *to* your partner to belonging *with* your partner. There is no question that you can survive without your partner; you are with your partner by choice.

THE COMMITTED SINGLE

People who choose to live alone or have relationships without a definite time commitment are not necessarily horizontal lovers. They are at peace living alone, and when they enter relationships they may or may not continue to live alone. Their relationships are called *serial commitments* because they commit to a partner instead of committing to longevity with a partner. Committed singles are usually happy and healthy. Rather than being based on fear of commitment, their choice to live alone is based on an honest, existential assessment of how they want to experience their personal journey. Most importantly, committed singles are loyal to the partner in their serial relationships and very honest about their intentions and expectations. So how do they differ from horizontal lovers?

The essential differences are based on approaching instead of avoiding life, and honesty in their propositions instead of manipulative hidden agendas. Committed singles live in peace within their solitude; horizontal lovers live in turbulence within their loneliness. With committed singles, what you see is what you get, and with horizontal lovers, what you get is what they want you to see.

It's important to identify the differences between committed singles and horizontal lovers to avoid pathological labels for healthy choices; in fact, I disagree with clinicians who categorically define serial commitments as one of the symptoms of commitment phobia. In my view, these clinicians are assuming you are psychologically flawed if you do not commit to a partner for life. On the contrary, I submit that you are emotionally healthy as long as you have worthy intentions and honest expectations when you enter a relationship—or choose to live alone. But I will admit there are many more horizontal lovers in the world than committed singles. And my advice to horizontal lovers is to differentiate between *fearing loneliness* and *loving solitude,* to identify who taught you to falsify who you are, to reclaim your sense of worthiness, and to allow love to teach you how to be honest with yourself and others. Then choose to be either a committed single or a vertical lover.

NAVIGATIONAL TOOLS FOR GUARDIANS OF THE HEART

Now it's time for direct experience of the lessons in this chapter.

When you were learning to walk, ride a bike, or drive a car, you had no guarantees of success before you started your lessons. Did you stop walking or riding your bike when you fell, or stop driving when you bumped into another car? Why not? Because increasing your *competence* gave you faith to continue without any guarantees. No fears, including the fear of emotional wounding, can be resolved with guarantees or appeals to logic. It does not follow, however, that their solutions are uncertain or illogical. As I do with most biocognitive lessons, in this section, I will use the principles of incidental learning to teach you how to resolve your fear of future wounds—if that is your issue. If you do not have that fear, you can still apply incidental learning to other challenges in your relationship.

Let me reiterate how I define incidental learning. In the process of learning a given task, you coincidentally gain competence in something else. Examples abound: children play video games and incidentally learn eye-motor coordination, we dance and incidentally learn balance, and when we practice tai chi, we incidentally learn focused attention. And, if you saw the original *Karate Kid,* you could wax a car using clockwise and counterclockwise motions and incidentally learn how to block punches.

You may recall that in chapter 2, I explained how changing your felt meaning takes place at the interaction of field horizons. In the following exercises, you will experience shifting from your field of fear to your field of competence. Felt meaning is recontextualized in the gap between field horizons. Remember: you don't have to have epiphanies or intellectual understanding to recontextualize felt meaning. It happens incidentally.

◇◇◇◇◇◇◇◇◇◇◇◇◇◇◇◇◇◇◇◇◇◇◇◇◇◇◇◇◇◇◇◇◇◇◇◇◇

Incidental Lessons to Resolve
Your Fear of Being Wounded Again

Practice each of the following steps for a few minutes. You can read the instructions through a few times before doing each step with your eyes closed, or with your eyes open. You can also return to this exercise anytime you need more practice. When you assimilate the principles you learn, they will become natural strategies to navigate your relationship with yourself and others.

❖ To *incidentally* relax, sit comfortably in a quiet place
   and *observe* the flow of sensations, emotions, and
   thoughts in your mindbody.

❖ Recall memories of riding your bike after you learned
   balance, solving multiplication problems after you

learned arithmetic, and any other memories of
reaching competence.

❖ Embody your competency memories and pay attention
to your mindbody manifestations.

❖ Although you may not remember how you learned a
task, you remember the competence you achieved.

❖ Repeat the following words in your mind,
"Competence reduces fear." As you repeat them like
a mantra, observe how your mindbody responds.
Rather than interpreting the words, experience
the felt meaning of the words. (Felt meaning is
the mindbody experience that words, phrases, and
symbols elicit in you.)

❖ Repeat the following words, "Competence *does not*
reduce fear." As you repeat the phrase like a mantra,
observe how your mindbody responds. Rather than
interpreting the words, experience the felt meaning of
the phrase.

❖ After repeating "Competence does not reduce fear" a
few times, repeat, "Competence reduces fear" a few
times. Experience the felt meaning of each mantra.

❖ Continue shifting from one mantra to the other and
notice differences in their felt meaning.

❖ When you shift from one mantra to the other, observe
the gap between shifts. Experience the felt meaning
of the gap. The felt meaning can also be the *void of
experience* in the gap. Do not set expectations.

❖ Slowly count from one to five and open your eyes.
   Reorient yourself to your surroundings before
   getting up.

To solidify what you learned in this exercise, the next time you
experience fear of being wounded again in your relationship,
focus on the competence you need at that moment to reduce
your fear. Shift from the felt meaning of your fear to the
felt meaning of the competence you need to reduce your
fear. Repeat the shifts for a few minutes as you did in this
contemplative exercise. When you identify the competence you
need, apply it and practice it in other circumstances as well.

For example, let's say your partner disappoints you by
forgetting a special date, and your fear surfaces. Without
suppressing the felt meaning the fear elicits, what can you
do to gain competence in dealing with your disappointment?
You could learn to discern the differences in contexts where
this fear surfaces; you realize that you feel more fear when
your partner forgets your anniversary than when your partner
forgets to reserve tickets for a play. Recognizing this now,
you could learn to express to your partner what you expect
on special dates, explaining how important celebrating
your anniversary is to you. You could learn to express your
disappointment without playing the victim, perhaps by
allowing that occasional forgetting is understandable, but a
habitual pattern of forgetting is not. You could even learn to
celebrate a forgotten special date by celebrating the anniversary
at another time.

The exercises you learn indirectly reduce your fear of
being wounded by incidentally increasing your faith in the
relationship while you are learning ways to become competent.
In other words, faith is what inspires us to proceed without
any evidence of the outcome we expect. We will use *faith in
the outcome* in the next exercise.

Identifying Your Stage of Vertical Love

The exercise in this section will teach you how to identify the stage at which you are experiencing vertical love.

* To *incidentally* relax, sit comfortably in a quiet place and *observe* the flow of sensations, emotions, and thoughts in your mindbody. You can close your eyes or keep them open.

* Ask yourself the following question, answering it with complete honesty, "Do I *mostly* feel my partner is still my friend, or has our friendship weakened or disappeared?" Here you are assessing the *attraction stage*.

* Based on your answer, experience the felt meaning of *still my friend* or *no longer my friend.*

* If you have the relationship you want, shift from the felt meaning of what you have to the felt meaning of how you can celebrate what you have.

* Ask yourself the following question, answering it with complete honesty, "Do I *mostly* have a ledger relationship based on compromise, a win-win relationship based on finding common ground, or a belonging-without-ownership relationship that supports our respective joy fingerprints?" Here, you're assessing the *engagement stage*.

* Based on your answer, experience the felt meaning of the relationship you have.

* If you have the relationship you want, shift from what you have to how you can celebrate what you have.

❖ Ask yourself the following question, answering it with complete honesty, "Is my relationship *mostly* a fusion of the best of our individual histories, the worst of our individual histories, or domination of one history over the other?" Here you're considering the *engagement stage.*

❖ Based on your answer, experience the felt meaning of the relationship you have.

❖ If you have the relationship you want, shift from what you have to how you can celebrate what you have.

If you have identified your stage and the progress you want to make, go to the next exercise. If you are not clear on where you are in the stages, practice the preceding exercise as needed before moving to the next.

Improving and Transitioning Your Stage of Vertical Love

The previous exercise helped you identify the stage that best describes your vertical love. Use that stage as a starting place for this next exercise, which will teach you how to progress within this stage. You can go back to regain what may be missing, improve where you are, or progress to the next stage. If you and your partner are joyfully living in stage three, use this exercise to help you identify ways to celebrate your accomplishments.

❖ To *incidentally* relax, sit comfortably in a quiet place and *observe* the flow of sensations, emotions, and thoughts in your mindbody. You can close your eyes or keep them open.

❖ Determine whether you want to improve your present stage, return to a previous stage, or progress to another stage.

❖ Based on your decision, identify what is lacking and what you require to improve your competence in that area. Experience the felt meaning of what you identify.

❖ Recall times when you committed to improving something in your life without having faith in the outcome you wanted. Perhaps you started to exercise regularly but had no clear idea of the results you might expect, or you started a savings account with an unclear idea of how much you might save. Experience the felt meaning of your commitment.

❖ Experience the felt meaning of your doubts about the outcome: what it felt like to have only a vague idea of what it might be like to be more physically fit, or to have a little money put away.

❖ Experience the felt meaning of what you accomplished without having faith in the outcome: noticing that your clothes fit differently, or that you felt more secure with a little money in the bank.

❖ Imagine you are doing what you have determined is necessary to remain in, return to, or transition your stage of vertical love. Experience the felt meaning of doing it without faith in your desired outcome.

❖ Experience what you feel when you advance without evidence to confirm you will reach your goal. Experience other memories of commitments without evidence. The felt meaning of what you are experiencing is your faith! Faith in yourself.

❖ Before you count from one to five to conclude this exercise, commit to look for instances in your relationship in which you advance without evidence.

◇◇◇

Breaking Through Your Novelty Plateaus

To avoid running from or enduring boring reruns, the next exercise will teach you effective methods to break through novelty plateaus. In the exercise, I will use *biocognitive iteration* and a concept I modified from Buddhism that I call *novelty kindness*. In Buddhist philosophy, the term is *lovingkindness:* one of the *four immeasurables.* In chapter 9, I will explain the Buddhist four immeasurables and their applications to biocognitive science, but for our purposes here, novelty kindness means kindness that is drawn from love and can be used to find the novelty in boring reruns. This is a key to shifting out of novelty plateaus and letting creativity fly.

❖ To *incidentally* relax, sit comfortably in a quiet place and *observe* the flow of sensations, emotions, and thoughts in your mindbody. You can close your eyes or keep them open.

❖ Identify a boring rerun you use with your partner and experience its felt meaning. For example, reciting the same line from a movie you enjoyed together whenever a certain situation arises, or repeating a joke whose punch line has gone flat.

❖ Recall the original function of the rerun and experience its felt meaning. The initial function could be to share humor, give a warning, express dissatisfaction with your partner, a rerun you learned from cultural editors, and so on.

❖ Identify a boring rerun of your partner's and experience its felt meaning. For example, coming home and going to the laptop instead of stopping for a hug and kiss. Recall the original function of the rerun and experience its felt meaning. The initial function could be humor, a warning, an expression of dissatisfaction with your partner, a rerun learned from cultural editors, and so on.

❖ Imagine your partner engaged in the rerun, and allow yourself to feel the usual emotional reaction you have.

❖ Recall a loving memory of something your partner did with you or for you. Experience the felt meaning of the memory.

❖ Now recall your partner's rerun again and experience its felt meaning. Bring your felt meaning of the loving experience to awareness.

❖ Shift between the felt meaning of your partner's rerun and the loving experience.

❖ After shifting the two felt meanings, allow the loving felt meaning to grow, and begin to look for ways of discovering a new meaning in the routine.

❖ Experience new ways of interpreting the rerun and a message it could carry that you have not been heeding. For example, if your partner repeats a vague criticism when you sit for dinner, look for messages the rerun may carry that you have not been willing to hear: you are drinking too much, you're not giving me enough attention, you're not taking care of yourself, you've been ridiculing me in public, and so on.

❖ Before ending this exercise, commit to responding to your own novelty plateaus or your partner's with novelty kindness: drawing from love to find novelty and unheard messages in reruns.

❖ Count from one to five, open your eyes, and reorient yourself before getting up.

In addition to signaling a need for fresh information, novelty plateaus have another function: to convey unheard messages. They can be a plea to be heard, to be understood. The boring repetition that a stormy morning is an opportunity to dance in the rain may be a message from your partner that your relationship needs a new dance. Nothing is expressed without function, and no one enjoys being boring!

❖ ❖ ❖

In this chapter you learned ways to create or improve your relationship with your partner, yourself, your God, or whomever else you choose to share your journey with. In the next chapter we will investigate a new topic: moving from joyful relationships to healthy longevity.

Lessons from Centenarians

ONE HUNDRED YEARS YOUNG

Growing older is a natural process we all experience. *Aging,* on the other hand, is a dysfunctional concept: an assimilation of cultural portals that define how our biology "should" respond to the passing of time. I have done extensive research with healthy centenarians (100 years or older) in varied cultures. This chapter, based on what I discovered, addresses the common traits, beliefs, and concepts of aging that contribute to the wellness and longevity of the longest-living people in the world. In it, I will share with you ways you can modify "aging consciousness" in a society that does not support growing older for what it is: an opportunity to increase your value and competence.

One of my paradoxical findings is that, when centenarians reach the more infrequent level of longevity called *supercentenarians* (110 years or older), the rate of deleterious aging effects actually diminishes. Although there are only a few hundred verified living supercentenarians—90 percent of whom are women—I propose that one of the reasons for their extended healthy longevity is that they have had more time to practice the things that cause health!

CULTURAL PORTALS

Cultural portals convey powerful warnings that we are to maintain collective identity and tribal control. Admonitions such as "You are too old for that" or "What do you expect at your age?" define the horizons of the elderly portal and determine how you are expected to perceive the world within that perspective. These warnings are hypnotic, and they restrict your options in life and control the rate of your biological aging. Growing older is the mindbody passing through time and space, whereas *aging* is the mindbody's response to the cultural limitations it assimilates.

Fortunately, centenarians all over the world defy disempowering cultural portals and show us that resilient subcultural beliefs, rather than genetics, are some of the most important contributors to their longevity. They come from cultures whose tribal beliefs are not unlike those I suggest contribute to aging. But their conviction to question what does not personally make sense to them liberates them from tribal constraints; they choose healthy defiance of the tribe where others opt for unhealthy compliance with it. Toxic lessons from cultural editors have a limited effect on centenarians because they learned early in life to imagine a world beyond the one their culture narrowly defines. When you meet healthy centenarians, you realize they don't fit the stereotype of their age.

CULTURAL TIME

According to biocognitive theory, *cultural time* comprises the attributions, rituals, admonitions, beliefs, and other horizons we interweave into the time and space of our *embodied perception*. While *growing older* only requires the passing of time, *aging* is significantly affected by the cultural history we embody. Biology is sculpted within the cultural portals we choose to enter, and healthy longevity is enhanced by the resilience we learn from our challenges. It is essential to recognize *time* as an invention we devised to measure our movement through space. Our primal ancestors lived in the immediate present without conception of past and future. The capacity to build tools indicates an ability to plan for the future: making things to use in the present, planning to reuse them in the future, and recalling having made them in the past. Although we have progressed more than seventy thousand years since our species discovered past and future, we continue to see time as something more than an artifact to measure our movement in space. Just as we define our work and rest space in segments of seven days, we determine youngness and oldness in segments of years—segments that are culturally defined, not biologically determined. For example, seventy is the new fifty, and in Roman times thirty was old age. So . . . does time age us, or do our cultures tell us what we should do with our time? I will show you how to navigate your space using centenarian conception of time.

HEALTHY DEFIANCE OF CULTURAL EDITORS

We learn valuable lessons from our cultural editors, some painful and some loving. But whether they are unpleasant or joyful, we *must* choose what to incorporate and discard from those lessons when we move beyond accepted culture. We learn some of our most useful lessons under very turbulent conditions. Thus, feeling good or bad while learning lessons is not what determines their quality or usefulness; it is the honor, commitment, and loyalty we extract from them that defines these. This distinction can help us decide which messages from our cultural editors we should righteously defy and which we should gratefully assimilate.

The centenarians I've investigated seem to have had an instinctive ability to discern early in life which lessons from their cultural editors they must deeply question and ultimately defy. In fact, although some centenarians I have met had horrendous cultural editors, they were always able to recall someone who, however briefly, stepped into their misery to offer them a gift of love.

What is the lesson here? To realize, independent of the hell we may have gone through, that deep in our memories there are forgotten gifts of random kindness that we neglected to assimilate. Finding those forgotten gifts can be an impetus for resilience.

A patient I was treating for post-traumatic stress disorder could not recall a single act of kindness from her past. After she related her childhood memories, it was not difficult to understand why she was stuck in her infernal present. Her father had sexually abused her from the age of five until she ran away from home at fifteen. When other children were happily anticipating arriving home from school to a cozy environment, my patient was trying to figure out how to avoid her despicable father's sexual abuse. I could not get a single pleasant memory out of her.

After weeks of practicing a contemplative technique I taught her, she was able to identify an act of kindness in her life. One cold and snowy afternoon, she was walking home from school with her usual apprehension, and an elderly lady who lived a few houses away signaled her to approach. The kind woman asked her to come in from the snow and offered her freshly baked cookies and hot chocolate! I will admit that when my patient finished her story, I defied a stupid rule prohibiting psychologists from touching their patients. I held her in my arms, and we both cried. It was soon after that act of kindness that my patient ran away from home.

What does this compelling story have to do with centenarians and their longevity? It encapsulates the essence of healthy defiance. Before we can righteously defy, we have to feel *worthy* of defying. And when we defy malevolence, we can find our freedom. Centenarians instinctively know that such random acts of kindness form the foundation of their resilience. Independent of their emotional storms, they can always recall memories of compassion from their past.

CENTENARIAN MINDFULNESS

Resilience, perseverance, creativity, and flexibility are all attributes I have found in every healthy centenarian I have studied, in cultures spanning five continents. Fortunately, we can learn all of these attributes without relying on our genetic endowment or family history. There are no genes we can isolate to identify the centenarian mind, but we can learn the characteristics that contribute to longevity if we shift our own mindset from one of *passing time* to one of *engaging space*. What do I mean by this existential challenge? We need to snap out of our hypnotic concept of time in which *things happen to us* in sequence, and instead be mindful of how *we can happen in our space* without assigning a sequence. I will clarify with a few examples.

It's Monday morning, and your car won't start. You call a taxi so you can get to work, and it takes forty-five minutes to arrive. When you finally get to work, you realize you have forgotten to mail an important report to a client. That "sequence" of turbulent events begs to be connected using *cognitive strings* that only exist in your mind: what a horrible start to the week! We impose sequence to our time so we can make sense of the space we travel. But since we tie sequence with cognitive strings to events in our time/space, we are equally capable of untying them with the attributes centenarians share: the *creativity* to reinterpret negative attributions, the *flexibility* to consider other options, the *perseverance* to endure turbulence, and the *resilience* to engage new mindsets.

Let me further clarify. Although we need to form cognitive strings in order to make sense of our world, when faced with the kinds of circumstances I have just described, we impose a sequence to unrelated events that creates false cause and effect. Your car not starting and your forgetting to mail a report have no cause-and-effect link, but if you tie them together with cognitive strings, you may conclude that everything is going wrong for you that day—that it has been going wrong and will continue to deteriorate. Conversely, crashing your car because your brakes are bad or missing a flight because your connection was delayed have external cause and effect. Although you could conclude from both sets of circumstances that your day is not going well, in one set of events you created false cause and effect—these things are happening because I'm having a bad day—and in the other the cause and effect are demonstrably clear.

Toward the end of the chapter, I will show you how to incorporate the centenarian attributes that can free you from the deleterious effects of creating false cause and effect. For now, just entertain the notion that sequence lives in your mind, and begin to notice how many of your conclusions about your life events are based on how you have learned to group your experiences together.

THE SEMANTIC SPACE OF CULTURAL PORTALS

In biocognitive practice, I adapt Charles Osgood's concept of *semantic differential* and apply it to describing cultural portals. Osgood was a psychologist who, along with his colleagues George Suci and Percy

Tannenbaum, investigated how to measure semantic meaning. They found that humans across cultures give linguistic meaning to their experiences using three semantic dimensions: *evaluation, potency,* and *activity.* Each of these semantic dimensions has pairs of opposite adjectives to describe objects, people, concepts, and ideas. For example, evaluation includes opposite pairs of adjectives such as good-bad, pretty-ugly, happy-sad. Potency includes strong-weak, powerful-powerless, rugged-delicate. Activity includes fast-slow, active-passive, alert-drowsy. In other words, without being aware of it, when we describe what we perceive, we categorize using language based on opposite adjectives that define value, strength, and movement.

How does semantic differential apply to cultural portals? Since our language affords us three categories with which to define our experiences, we can identify the semantic space a culture determines for each portal. But just as we are not aware of how cultural editors influence our sense of value or worth, we enter cultural portals without recognizing how their semantic space molds our conduct and expectations.

In the biocognitive model, infancy, childhood, adolescence, young adulthood, middle age, and old age are portals with culturally defined semantic spaces. For example, most cultures predominantly categorize the infancy portal as follows: evaluation—cute, adorable, and innocent; potency—weak and defenseless; and activity—slow and passive. Imagine moving from portal to portal in your culture without realizing the programming that's taking place. The valuation, potency, and activity assigned to each portal is culturally defined rather than biologically determined.

For our purpose, let's concentrate on centenarians and the semantic space they construct for their portals. While Western cultures tend to conclude that value, potency, and activity decrease with age, centenarians do not buy into this proposition; they view their journey through life quite differently. Rather than diminish their value, potency, and activity, they increase their *worthiness, complexity,* and *passion.* Not surrendering to culturally determined portals is the most powerful contributing factor to their longevity. And again, what they do intuitively, you can learn to do mindfully!

FOUR COMMITMENTS FOR
CENTENARIAN MINDFULNESS

My investigation of centenarians has taught me that these people share four essential beliefs. If we commit to learning and assimilating them, we can increase our own healthy longevity.

1 Growing older is the passing of time; aging is what we do with time based on our cultural beliefs.

2 The present moment is never too late to make commitments.

3 Illnesses are learned; the causes of health are inherited.

4 Forgiveness is a liberating act of self-love.

As I identified the beliefs that centenarians from different cultures share, a very interesting pattern emerged. Although there were differences in language, folklore, diet, socioeconomics, politics, and religion, I discovered there is something I now call *centenarian mindfulness,* finding novelty and wisdom in the challenges one encounters. I'll give you a few examples:

❖ Being in a concentration camp, learning to enjoy small amounts of deplorable food, realizing how much we overeat, and learning to transform isolation into contemplative solitude.
❖ After losing both parents early in life, discovering fatherly and motherly qualities within and using them to guide personal development.
❖ Mourning the death of a spouse by celebrating the privilege of having shared a loving journey.
❖ Forgiving an act of malevolence, thereby taking back the power given to the perpetrator.

I could go on indefinitely with further examples, but you get the essence of the freshness and wisdom centenarians possess. I must emphasize, however, that these experiences did not result from naive "positive thinking." Centenarians experience the depth of their pain, but they also know how to access personal power to learn from their pain. I am reminded, although Nietzsche is one of my favorite existentialist philosophers, that his dictum "what does not kill you makes you stronger" needs modification, especially since it did not work very well for him. Remember, he attempted suicide several times. If you take his statement literally, you might conclude that pain is your only teacher. Most important, what centenarian mindfulness can contribute to Nietzsche's proposal is this: you must not remain in your hell. Thus, a Nietzschean centenarian would add, "if you find the wisdom to relinquish your pain."

Now let's return to the four commitments. Toward the end of the chapter, I'll show you how to gradually incorporate each of them into your life.

First Commitment

Growing older is the passing of time; aging is what we do with time based on our cultural beliefs.

By now you know I repeat new concepts throughout the book because, as I explained in chapter 4, this biocognitive iteration means that each repetition adds new information to expand and deepen your felt meaning of a new concept. I've also shown the difference between aging and growing older, but what may need demonstration is how centenarians intuitively *live* the difference, and how they defy cultural editors who attempt to dissuade them from their individualism.

While most people progressively slow down, become less curious, and assume that their abilities will diminish as they age, centenarians do not follow this pattern. Instead, the semantic space of their cultural portal increases in complexity and new learning. When you ask them what their plans are for the future, their answers describe a future you might associate with someone forty years younger. Here are a few actual examples from my field notes of how centenarians conceptualize their existence in time and space:

MARIO "I like your vegetable garden. Tell me about it."

101-YEAR-OLD MAN "I love the way it's turning out, but wait till you see it in three or four years."

MARIO "I was told you lost your sight last year. How are you adjusting?"
102-YEAR-OLD MAN "I was sad for a while, but now when I talk to a woman, I have to touch her to know who she is." (Rascally smile when he tells me.)

MARIO "I understand you have a new love in your life."
100-YEAR-OLD WOMAN "Yes, I like younger men, so I got me an eighty-year-old beau who writes me poems."

MARIO "When was the last time you went to a doctor?"
100-YEAR-OLD MAN "A long time ago. At least thirty years."
MARIO "And what do your doctors have to say about that?"
100-YEAR-OLD MAN "I don't know—they're all dead."

These fascinating responses illustrate centenarian mindfulness of the first commitment. They defy tribal conventions of time, disregard the admonishments of authorities, and inhabit a space that defies the stereotypes of aging.

Please know that I am not advocating you avoid health care professionals, I am simply reporting what seems to work for some centenarians. Modern medicine has much to offer, as long as you avoid predatory doctors, those who sell fear more than healing.

Second Commitment

The present moment is never too late to make commitments.

In addition to molding how you age, cultural portals define how you are supposed to plan your future. In most cultures, the young adult portal is very different from the old age portal. For example, you may be praised if you decide to go to college at thirty, but if you make that same decision at eighty, you will most likely encounter killjoy comments such as "At your age?" and "Take it easy and enjoy your retirement." Your well-meaning friends are not aware they are living in the semantic space of a portal they bought from their culture rather than exploring the opportunities life has to offer them at any age. The following responses to my questions are examples of the second mindfulness commitment: it's never too late to engage your passion.

MARIO "Do you have any plans for this year?"

103-YEAR-OLD MAN "Yes—I am taking tango lessons. I always wanted to learn in Buenos Aires, but with the money I'm saving by taking lessons here in town instead, I'll be able to do other fun things."

MARIO "Your friend tells me you're getting married again."

105-YEAR-OLD MAN "Yeah, my girlfriend wants to start a family." (Raucous laughter after he says this.)

MARIO "And how old is your girlfriend?"

105-YEAR-OLD MAN "Well, she lies about her age, but I bet she's pushing ninety."

MARIO "You sprained your ankle jogging. Are you going to stop running?"

100-YEAR-OLD MAN "Yeah, sprains are hard to heal, but I joined a swimming team, and I am going to compete next year in my age group."

MARIO "And how many other swimmers are in your age group?"

100-YEAR-OLD MAN "These two other old guys who think they're great." (The two "old guys" were ninety and ninety-one.)

These amusing excerpts may seem made up, but I assure you, I had the best time hearing all the ways these exceptional people break patterns set by those who *think* old. For most centenarians, the present moment is never too late to make commitments. And the centenarian jogger illustrates another interesting characteristic I noticed in many male centenarians; they refer to other elderly men as "old guys." They also frequently tell you they don't like to be around "old people." Why? The most frequent answer I have heard is, "Old people are always complaining about their aches and pains." I was amused to learn most of these "old people" are much younger than the centenarians who avoid them. And here is another centenarian insight: many view themselves as significantly younger than their age.

Your lesson here is clear: don't ever let anyone kill your dreams because of the quantity of life-space you have traveled. Let the fearful call it their time, and you can call it your space.

Third Commitment

Illnesses are learned; the causes of health are inherited.

In chapter 3, I explained the science that underlies how, based on our cultural beliefs and life choices, we teach our nervous, immune, and endocrine systems to break down, as well as how our genes relentlessly express our inherited causes of health rather than sentencing us to inevitable illness. Now we can look at what centenarians have to say about their genetics—better yet, how they *live* their genetics.

MARIO "How old were your parents when they died?"
100-YEAR-OLD MAN "My dad was seventy, and my mother was eighty-one."

MARIO "Were either of your parents centenarians?"
101-YEAR-OLD WOMAN "No, my mother lived to be seventy-nine, and my father was around seventy-five when he passed."

MARIO "Do you have any relatives who were centenarians?"
103-YEAR-OLD MAN "What the hell is a centurion?"
MARIO "No, I said centenarians—people one hundred years or older."
103-YEAR-OLD MAN "Oh, well, I had a great-uncle who lived to be ninety-nine."

MARIO "What illnesses were most common in your family?"
106-YEAR-OLD WOMAN "I think cancer and diabetes."

MARIO "Do you have any illnesses?"
106-YEAR-OLD WOMAN "I got a little arthritis and can't hear too good."

MARIO "Did you know they call people your age supercentenarians?"
110-YEAR-OLD WOMAN "Really? I never thought I'd live this long."
MARIO "Have you noticed any change in your health the last couple of years?"
110-YEAR-OLD WOMAN "Not much. If I keep going like this, who knows how long I'll be around."

MARIO "Tell me about your diet. What types of food do you usually eat?"
100-YEAR-OLD WOMAN "I don't diet. I eat whatever I want. Some meat, some fried chicken, some fruit."

These answers reflect what I argue about healthy longevity. It is not primarily genetic endowment. Rather than inheriting illnesses, we are genetically predisposed to maintaining good health! But notice how these centenarians are not *trying* to live a long time. It is how they think and live that accounts for their longevity. I also found that their longevity is not so much about what they eat but how moderate they are with their eating. I'll have more to say about dining rituals later.

Fourth Commitment

Forgiveness is a liberating act of self-love.

This particular commitment to centenarian mindfulness is one of the most important. If you are reluctant to forgive, you relinquish your power to your perpetrator. Centenarians I studied consistently showed me they do not hold grudges. Let me illustrate with more excerpts from my field notes:

MARIO "You were in a concentration camp during World War II. How did you deal with it after you were freed?"

101-YEAR-OLD MAN "It was the worst experience in my life, but you know what I remember most? I was worried my mother wouldn't understand that they didn't let me write her." (He laughs about his concern.)

MARIO "So what did you do when you were freed?"

101-YEAR-OLD MAN "The first thing I did was to explain to my mother that the camp guards didn't allow mail. Boy, did she get upset with the guards." (More laughter.)

MARIO "How did you feel about the guards? Did you resent them?"

101-YEAR-OLD MAN "Hell, yeah! They were sons of bitches. But you know, I felt sorry for one of them because he was just a kid, like me. He used to bring me some bread when he could sneak it in. You know, I got to like that kid. He was risking his life trying to help me!"

MARIO "Did you forgive them for all they did to you?"

101-YEAR-OLD MAN "You think I was going to waste my time resenting those bastards? I kept thinking how lucky I was to find a friend who was supposed to be my enemy."

MARIO "Your stepfather sexually molested you when you were a teenager. How did you deal with it?"

100-YEAR-OLD WOMAN "He didn't sexually molest me—he raped me! I don't like those highfalutin words when shit happens. But you're a cute doctor, so I'll give you a break." (She winks and smiles when she tells me this.)

MARIO "How did you deal with the rape? Did you tell your mom?"

100-YEAR-OLD WOMAN "Back then I was furious, but when I think about it now, it makes me laugh knowing what I did to him. I felt sorry for my mother because she loved that beast. So I never told her. But let me tell you what I did to the beast. One day, my mom went for groceries, and the beast was taking a nap. I got the biggest knife I could find in the kitchen, and I went to his room. I woke him up with a hard slap and pointed the knife to his throat. And here's the part

I really enjoyed. I told him, 'If you ever come near me again, I'll cut your balls off!'" (She laughs with gusto.)

MARIO "What did he do?"

100-YEAR-OLD WOMAN "He avoided me like the plague. A few months later, he left my mother for another woman. And I taught my three daughters to never take any crap from men!" (She laughs triumphantly again.)

MARIO "Did you forgive him?"

100-YEAR-OLD WOMAN "I don't know if I did, but when I used to think about what he did to me, I'd feel really good about what I did to him."

These conversations more than suffice to highlight the process of letting go: forgiveness as a liberating act of self-love. The male centenarian implicitly celebrated with gratitude the guardian angel he met in a pit of inhumanity. By allowing gratitude to reign over bitterness, he was able to recontextualize his resentment. By shedding the weight of his resentment, he reclaimed the humanity that had been stolen from him. The female centenarian regained empowerment she lost through a shaming condition when she responded with honorable courage—a valuable lesson she passed on to her daughters.

Notice how these centenarians deal with their anger? Rather than repressing it, they express it in relevant contexts—and they let it go. You may recall from chapter 3 that righteous anger, expressed in the appropriate context, is actually good for your health. In chapter 8, I'll teach you a mindbody method to forgive through liberation from self-entrapment. You'll also learn why forgiveness has to do with power given away to your perpetrator and how to reclaim it. But the lesson here is to recognize that forgiveness is not an intellectual process to resolve using logical reasoning. Why? Because the wound is lodged in your mindbody bioinformational field, not in your logical mind.

CRAFTING CENTENARIAN MINDFULNESS

Learning to incorporate how centenarians structure their world and travel their space requires patience and perseverance. Although centenarians are quite flexible, I found that their rituals are very important to them. Let's define *ritual* as it relates to centenarian wellness, and differentiate it from *routine* and *habit*.

In centenarian mindfulness, ritual is purposeful action that connects us with our individual and cultural identity: celebrating birthdays, prayer, breaking bread with family and friends, pilgrimages to venerable places, and other expressions of individual and cultural identity. In contrast, *routine is something we do regularly because we believe we have to do it:* personal hygiene, grocery shopping, dressing, and any other behavior repeated to maintain our social status quo. And *habit is something we do regularly because we believe we are not able to change or are not aware we are doing it:* overeating, lying, tardiness, unhealthy caretaking, or any other behavior we do helplessly or without awareness.

As you can see, rituals, habits, and routines can be good or bad as well as, under certain conditions, difficult to differentiate from one another. Because their definitions sometimes overlap, most people use them interchangeably. But rather than further confuse these terms, I will illustrate their differences to help you craft centenarian mindfulness. We can further differentiate their meaning when we add *intention* and *awareness* to our definition. Let's see what happens when we determine function, intention, and awareness for ritual, routine, and habit.

I mentioned earlier that breaking bread with others has a positive, buffering effect on stress and illness. In fact, breaking bread in good company is one of the most beneficial rituals we can learn from centenarians. We know breaking bread with family and friends has at least two positive functions: nourishment and merriment. When we share a meal, we are also aware that our intentions could be gratitude, sharing news, bonding, generosity, mutual exploration, and so on. With a ritual of celebrating your birthday, you are aware that the *function* is to mark another year from your birth and your *intention* is to honor the date of your birth.

Now let's analyze a typical routine: bathing. The function of bathing is personal hygiene. We are certainly aware of the hygiene function, and perhaps an intention to relax, sing in the shower, or clear our thoughts.

But habit is different from ritual and routine, in that we are usually not aware of its function and intention. For example, if you habitually clear your throat when you lie, you may not be aware that this action functions to distract you from your apprehension of getting caught, or from your intention to be dishonest for fear of showing who you really are. In other words, if you are asked why you celebrate your birthday (ritual) or bathe (routine), you can give reasonable answers, but if you are asked why you clear your throat when you lie (habit), you would most likely be clueless. And yes, there are times when function and intention are the same, but you will see later why it's important to look for circumstances when they differ.

If you stick with me through these apparently simplistic mental gymnastics, toward the end of the chapter, I'll show you how to evaluate your own rituals, routines, and habits to help you craft centenarian mindfulness. But more important, you'll learn how to increase mindfulness in your rituals and routines, and decrease mindlessness in your habits. Later, I'll also explain why rituals are experiences of full-time mindfulness; routines, part-time mindfulness; and habits, full-time mindlessness.

THE MIDDLE WAY IN CENTENARIAN MINDFULNESS

Most major religions and philosophies warn about excesses and the detrimental imbalances they cause. But the *middle way* concept I present here should not be confused with passivity, forced abstinence, or middle-of-the-road compromises. Instead, the middle way is *purposeful action to find benign balance.* Buddha defined the middle way as taking actions or having attitudes that promote happiness for oneself and others. Aristotle saw the middle way as a *golden mean,* where virtue is in the middle and vice at each extreme. In other words, both Eastern and Western philosophies agree: the middle way is worth pursuing if you want to be ethical and happy.

Centenarians offer the best examples I have found of living middle way mindfulness. While some centenarians are pleasantly plump, none are morbidly obese; some smoke cigars and drink alcoholic beverages, but none are addicts; some are religious, but none are religious fanatics. But the most important lesson I have gleaned from how they live is that they instinctively practice what Buddha and Aristotle prescribe for happiness. In other words, rather than feeling deprived of pleasure when they avoid excess, they find pleasure in their middle way: joyful choice rather than forced abstinence. Here are some examples from my field notes:

MARIO "Do you smoke cigarettes or cigars?"

101-YEAR-OLD MAN "I smoke a cigar every night before I go to bed."

MARIO "Do you smoke any other time?"

101-YEAR-OLD MAN "No, only at bedtime."

MARIO "Why only at bedtime?"

101-YEAR-OLD MAN "Because that's the time when I enjoy my cigar."

MARIO "How long have you been doing this?"

101-YEAR-OLD MAN "Let me think . . . ah, about seventy-five years."

See the difference between ritual, habit, and routine? This short conversation is a clear example of middle way centenarian mindfulness: smoking a cigar before bedtime is a ritual with a function of bringing closure to his day, his intention is to enjoy ending his day, and his purposeful action to find the middle way in his smoking.

As you can see, I am gradually unfolding the secrets of longevity hidden in centenarians' mindfulness and their middle way. But how can abstinence give us pleasure? To help me answer this legitimate question, let's look at what we know from psychology about freedom of choice.

Jack Brehm was an American psychologist who studied an interesting phenomenon: people assign greater value to options that are not available to them when they want them. For example, say you go shopping and find a blouse you like, but it's not available in your size—you now want it more. In his reactance theory, Brehm proposes that our psychological conception of freedom is based on the number of options available. But although it appears that we increase our perception of the value of a thing if it is not available, what truly gains value is the lost option: the loss of freedom to choose. The blouse did not become more valuable; losing the option to have the blouse is what makes it more desirable.

Joyful Choice versus Forced Abstinence

It may be easier to understand why we risk our lives to preserve our freedom than how we can find joy in abstaining from pleasurable excess. I propose the reason is that we equate abstinence with deprivation. Although some highly pleasurable conditions may be harmful, we still pursue them and conclude that the only way to avoid them is by painfully abstaining from them. This reasoning can explain why addictions and compulsions have such poor prognoses; it's not very enticing to replace the pleasures of cocaine and junk food with the misery of abstinence. Although some professionals, when treating addictions and other excessive behaviors, may use more palatable words such as "willpower" and "internal control," their methods continue to rely heavily on forced abstinence. This is semantic shuffling rather than paradigm shifting. But rather than simply criticizing what does not work well, I will once again draw from centenarian wisdom to provide some answers. And I will add what we know from the psychological research on forced abstinence.

We feel deprived when we abstain from something pleasurable. Based on what we know from reactance theory, deprivation across time increases our need for what we have abstained from. For example, if you have an eating disorder, the longer you abstain from eating your favorite ice cream, the higher your probability of gorging the next time you have your ice cream. Forced abstinence delays your excessive need for food instead of resolving it.

So what do centenarians do to deal with their excesses? They have *mindful rituals* rather than *mindless needs*. We only abuse what we mindlessly need, not what we mindfully love. When I tell my obese patients I am going to teach them to love food, they laugh and tell me they already love food too much. After I laugh with them, I show them how to mindfully recognize they need food to replace a deprivation of self-love. We never abuse what we *mindfully* love. Also, when we can't have what we abuse, we look for something else to abuse. Sound familiar? We stop abusing cigarettes, and we start abusing food. And yes, I know the argument about how decreased nicotine in your system increases fat storage. But that is one of the convenient arguments given to explain the physiology of addiction without understanding the psychology of forced abstinence.

Finding Joy in Middle Way Choices

The mindful middle way option is far from boring and restrictive. It is not a mechanical formula to compromise your pleasure, and it does not restrict your freedom of choice. And you don't have to spend years meditating in a cave to achieve competence in this middle way mindfulness. It is available immediately, and you don't have to engage it constantly. Toward the end of this chapter, I'll show you how to discover joy in the mindful middle way option, but now let's look deeper into what I mean by the term and how it could work for you.

Suppose you have an excessive relationship with food—and you love your beer. You decide you want to cut back on beer and bread. You go to a restaurant with a friend, and the waiter brings you freshly baked bread. Your friend orders a cold beer. The forced abstinence approach requires giving up the options of eating bread and drinking beer; and if you abstain, you will probably feel resentful for having to give up what you desire. The perceived value of bread and beer will rise. Abstinence also affects the quality of your breaking bread with your friend because you can see that he is enjoying the meal without any restraints. No wonder it's so damn hard to diet! The good news is that diets don't work in the long run; there are better ways to deal with excessive behavior. An eating disorder is a compulsion rather than an addiction, and it is not an illness. It is a culturally learned pattern to distract you from self-love. I will have more to say about this in chapter 10.

Now let's return to the restaurant example and see what we can do with the mindful middle way option. Rather than resentment at giving up your option to eat and drink what you desire, you can experience the turbulence that abstinence creates. In other words, since your excessive eating is distracting you from self-love, you can experience what you feel when you choose to avoid that distraction. Initially, it may not feel pleasant, but you're not looking for joy in this experience—joy will come later. After you experience what your excessive eating has been covering up, you can choose a middle way option between the two extremes of "all the bread and beer you desire" (giving in to your desire) and "no bread and beer at all" (abstaining altogether).

Both extremes are grounded in capitulation, surrender, and helplessness. In bright contrast, mindfully looking for the middle way carries with it endless possibilities: one beer and no bread, one piece of bread and no beer, one piece of bread with no butter, half a beer and no bread, and so on. More important, after you let yourself experience how your distraction feels in your mindbody, whatever middle way option you choose will be grounded in self-love.

In the process of choosing the middle way, you increase your *options* rather than your *resentment.* The middle way increases your sense of freedom, while forced abstinence decreases it.

PRACTICAL TOOLS FOR CENTENARIAN MINDFULNESS

As I've said, the practical exercises at the end of each chapter are designed to be incorporated gradually into your life. I suggest you return again and again to the practical methods in each chapter until you feel you can competently perform them. In this chapter, I'll show you how to turn centenarian concepts into centenarian mindfulness with tools for longevity.

◇◇

Determining Your Cultural Portals, Cultural Time, and Cultural Editors

❖ Find a quiet place to sit and calm your busy mindbody. Breathe slowly and observe what is going on in your mindbody and around you.

❖ Think of your age and determine whether you are in the cultural portal that is typical of your age. For example, are you complying with how you "should" dress, behave, and live?

❖ Have you changed your semantic space (conceptual meaning based on three dimensions): more or less value, activity, and power compared to your previous portal?

For example, if you are middle-aged, is your semantic space different from when you were a young adult? If you think of something you might like to change about your semantic space, bring it to the next exercise.

◇◇◇◇◇◇◇◇◇◇◇◇◇◇◇◇◇◇◇◇◇

Worthy Defiance

If you are happy with your present status, skip this exercise and go to the next. If you want to defy the cultural editors who influenced your compliance in how you are living in your present portal, continue with this exercise.

❖ Recall someone who confirmed your worthiness with acts of kindness and generosity, someone who recognized that you are special. Perhaps when you were very young, a teacher praised you for sharing your favorite toy with another child who had been sitting alone in a corner.

❖ Experience what you feel from this empowering memory and remember where and how you had this experience.

❖ When you want to defy any of the cultural editors who molded you into a portal and semantic space that you no longer want, bring back the mindbody experience of validation, and commit to changing that aspect of your life. Maybe you have been thinking about cutting back on exercise because you're getting on in years, and you don't want to do too much—you might strain your joints at this age.

❖ Any time you try to change but find resistance, from yourself or others, embody the experience of validation and do whatever you consider self-loving to implement change. In this example, walk an extra lap around your neighborhood on your daily walk. Notice how your body responds to your defiance. Simply observe whatever surfaces and let it pass.

❖ Allow your coauthors to not like your decision. They may not be ready to change when you are. Ignore the admonition, "Now be careful not to tire yourself out!"

❖ You can use the same exercise for any other worthy defiance. For example, you're too old to fall in love again, go back to college, or learn a new language.

◇◇◇◇◇◇◇◇◇◇◇◇◇◇◇◇◇◇◇◇◇◇◇◇◇◇◇◇◇◇◇◇◇◇

Cutting Cognitive Strings

❖ Recall a time when you had a bad day.

❖ Review all the negative details you can recall and determine whether you tied events together in a sequence in your mind to conclude that it was a bad day. If you did, recognize that it was your cognitive strings at work rather than real cause and effect.

❖ Observe what you feel when you recognize how you construct your day to be either good or bad.

❖ Next time you begin to have a "bad day," be mindful of how you may be using cognitive strings to create a cause-and-effect sequence that exists only in your mind.

❖ When you find false stringing like this, take a deep breath and celebrate that you are gaining centenarian wisdom.

◇◇◇◇◇◇◇◇◇◇◇◇◇◇◇◇◇◇◇◇◇◇◇◇◇◇◇◇◇◇◇◇◇◇◇

Four Commitments for Centenarian Mindfulness

* Decide which of the four commitments you want to incorporate in your life. Identify whom or what you have to defy. For example, ask yourself if you have bought into any of these myths: aging equals deterioration, it's too late to make commitments, you are sentenced to illness by your family history of illnesses, you can't forgive yourself or someone else. (If forgiveness is your issue, work on the other commitments now and address forgiveness after you read chapter 8.)

* Defying cultural editors is always done from valuation mindfulness. Embody your memory of being valued, and defy the editor, first using imagery, and then in real life. But remember, biocognitive defiance is not the same as confrontation.

* Rather than confronting your cultural editors from the past and your coauthors in the present, simply respond differently to their disempowering behavior. For example, in response to "Don't tire yourself out too much" you might say, "Thanks for your concern, but I'm not worried about getting tired. I'm walking to get stronger."

* Give your coauthors permission to not like your new response. If you are dealing with issues connected to someone who is no longer in your life, do the exercise using imagery, and embody both the apprehension and empowerment from the experience.

◇◇◇

Choosing Middle Way Mindfulness

❖ Identify a habit you want to change.

❖ Imagine you have given up what you are doing excessively; for example, having three beers at dinner.

❖ Imagine giving up the three beers and feel whatever happens when you abstain. Identify what you're avoiding by indulging; it might be anxiety or open, honest dialogue during dinner. Maybe you have been avoiding a long-overdue conversation about parenting your teenager, or sharing your worries about finances.

❖ Experience the avoidance in your mindbody and observe what happens without trying to change it.

❖ Let what you feel be your first step toward middle way mindfulness and enjoy the achievement, as small as it may feel.

❖ After facing your avoidance, commit to resolving what you have been avoiding without the beer. For example, if it's anxiety, identify the feeling throughout the day and use a relaxation technique to replace the avoidance.

❖ Now that you are aware of your avoidance, return to what you used as the avoidance: the three beers at dinner.

❖ Envision the two extremes. For example, no beer at all at one extreme and ten beers at the other. Generate middle way options: one beer per meal, one beer every other meal, half a bottle with your meal, bottled water instead of bottled beer, one beer during honest conversation, and so on.

❖ Experience what you feel when you create all
your options, and sense that you are increasing
your freedom rather than your deprivation.

❖ From your mindbody sense of increased
freedom, choose your middle way option from
all the options you have generated.

❖ Enjoy your middle way choice free of guilt
and resentment.

❖ Apply middle way mindfulness to any other
habits you want to change.

❖ ❖ ❖

I hope you have gleaned from this chapter that longevity is mostly
learned and that habits are fed by mindlessness and changed by the
middle way mindfulness centenarians naturally adopt. I will leave you
with a quote from Ellen Langer, my colleague and good friend, considered *the mother of mindfulness:* "Most suffering is a direct or indirect
result of mindlessness."

Abundance Phobia and Reclaiming Your Birthright of Wealth, Health, and Love

Fear of success is reaching pandemic proportions in prosperous societies today. We are taught to hide our personal excellence and to accept compliments only reluctantly. Although these cultural mandates to conceal our gifts and brush aside praise are intended to prevent an image of conceit, they compel us to learn a kind of false humility that does not serve us well in our relationships or in sustaining wellness.

This chapter offers practices to counter the cultural biases at the root of this problem. Drawing for this chapter on my work with celebrities, billionaires, and world leaders, I will share with you what I have learned about how cultural collectivism punishes individual excellence. I believe a lack of understanding of the anthropology underlying our tribal admonitions is a primary reason why many highly accomplished people coauthor their own self-destruction after they have achieved their desired goals.

CEILINGS OF ABUNDANCE

Our cultures determine the limits of acceptable individual achievements in wealth, health, and love—the three components of abundance. And they impose consequences for violating those limits by inflicting the wounds of abandonment, betrayal, and shame.

To examine the origin of these limits, we can turn to human history. Early tribal cultures enclosed their members' dwellings within fences or walls to protect against wild animals and enemies, containing them within the pale. The word *pale* is defined as "the limits within which one is privileged or protected." If you remained within the enclosure, within the pale, you were kept safe, you were accepted, and you were required to work for the collective benefit of the tribe. But if you went "beyond the pale," you were no longer considered a contributor to the tribe—venturing forth for your own benefit did not serve tribal needs.

With deep roots such as these, our modern cultures still teach us how far we can go on our paths to abundance, and the archetypal wounds they will inflict to keep us within the pale.

I had a patient who became a country music superstar in a very short period of time. He had grown up in a small town in rural Mississippi, and his family and community were very poor. He decided to go beyond the pale to find fame and fortune in Nashville, the mecca of country music.

At first, when he returned home for short visits, he was hailed as the town hero who had attained fame and abundance. But since *our collective psyche is still tribal,* his home visits became progressively more painful as his family and friends shifted their stance from admiration to resentment. They became envious of the superstar whom they now thought "was too good for his own good."

My patient had two choices: to remain beyond the pale with his new-found abundance and accept being banished emotionally from the tribe, or acquiesce to the tribe's collective needs and give up his abundance. He chose alcohol abuse as his ticket back to his known misery within the pale. Within a few months, he had lost all his money, property, and recording contracts.

Fortunately, he came to see me before completely deciding to give up and return to the tribe as a failure so he could be accepted again. After he learned to apply biocognitive tools, he was able to regain his abundance and understand that banishment was a limitation of his tribe rather than a curse.

By the way, he is no longer an "alcoholic" and enjoys fine wines with his meals. Although I agree that some people with alcohol challenges cannot be social drinkers, in chapter 10, I will explain why I believe addictions are sociocultural distractions to avoid worthiness, not diseases.

VENTURING BEYOND THE PALE

Abundance is usually a double-edged sword, because it brings joy at the price of banishment by the cultural editors who set ceilings for our achievements. But in biocognition, we study the successful outliers who have learned to venture beyond the pale without paying the tribal price. One of the ways you can begin to explore uncompromised abundance is to observe the conduct of people in your private and public life who are successful and healthy, because health is an expression of guilt-free abundance. But abundance does not mean perfect health, wealth, and love. Abundance is the waves of joy you can experience while sailing an imperfect ocean. Rather than help you search for a permanent state of bliss, I am going to show you how to navigate uncertainty with imperfection as your guide. These concepts may sound more poetic than practical, but I invite you to explore a path that will allow you to venture beyond the pale without sustaining personal damage. In this endeavor, my job is to provide you with the proper tools, and yours is to apply them with commitment.

ON A PATH TO ABUNDANCE

I propose that abundance is not sustainable without a strong sense of self-worth. Why not? Because maintaining health, reaching wealth, and finding love require the capacity to accept that you are worthy of your good fortune.

The limitations we learn from our cultures are embodied in our biology, determined for the individual by the collective consciousness of the group. A new condition that defies the established limits (horizons) of a bioinformational field causes turbulence, and puts pressure on the culture to assimilate or reject new information. When the train was invented, for example, it violated the established limit on speed that was based on how fast you could travel on horseback or by stagecoach. The train could reach an inconceivable speed of thirty-five miles per hour! The shakeup of that bioinformational field—the collective belief about speed—resulted in an ailment diagnosed as "railway spine" in travelers who experienced lumbar pain. When Otis invented the elevator, some users had nosebleeds after riding the innovative contraption that defied the familiar stairs. When airplanes were first commercialized, the vomit bag was a necessity for travel in those loud metal-winged tubes. Fortunately, belief horizons expand when the cultural collective consciousness assimilates new technology that has violated previous concepts of time and space.

You might ask what these advances in technology have to do with self-worthiness. The answer is that, in addition to enabling us to accept abundance with grace, self-worthiness also facilitates assimilating innovations that contribute to the quality of our lives. Why? Because we have to feel worthy before we can gracefully accept any new comfort or good fortune. Self-worthiness allows us to explore paths that lead to well-being and joy. Conversely, unworthiness is based on fear and devaluation, which limit our chances to reach abundance. Recall people you may know who live in fear, and you will find that deprivation, poor health, and failure are their way of life. Attempting to reach abundance without feeling worthy of accepting it is self-defeating; you will believe that abundance would never last because you don't deserve it—so why reach? And it is important to understand that self-defeating beliefs such as these are not conscious thoughts. They are hidden in the mindbody code you learned to keep you within the pale.

THE CHALLENGES OF SELF-WORTHINESS

If we must feel self-worthiness in order to gracefully accept good fortune, but our cultural editors taught us to devalue ourselves, are we sentenced to a life of failure? I strongly argue that, although it's not an easy task, anything we learned can be unlearned (recontextualized with new meaning). But before we attempt to unlearn what does not serve us well, we must also learn how to neutralize the tendency we have to sabotage ourselves on our journey to abundance.

Consider self-sabotage as your own attempts to keep *yourself* within the pale, and consider that it's your birthright to go beyond the pale. Also consider that expanding your ceilings of abundance sets an example of excellence for others to emulate; your success can be a gift of hope. But as is always the case when working with the mindbody code, these considerations need to be experienced (embodied) rather than intellectualized. If you imagine my suggestions without experiencing how your body and its sensations, emotions, and memories respond to the imagery, you will not reach the mindbody code of self-sabotage, and you must reach it in order to unlearn it. At the end of the chapter, I will teach you techniques to embody what you want to unlearn and relearn.

For now, let's continue with the conceptual implications of what we are trying to achieve. I propose that self-worthiness is a cultural interpretation constructed with horizons that determine how much abundance we can comfortably handle. We assimilate cultural interpretations based on the value our cultural editors determine and the level of abundance we are allowed to have without violating tribal horizons.

I should clarify that I am not suggesting that we are passive recipients of everything the cultural editors tell us about ourselves. Especially during adolescence, we tend to rebel against most tribal rules, and we attempt to define our own worthiness. Developmentally, this stage is very important because it helps us balance what we were told we are with what we experience on our own. But since our cultural editors are powerful figures in our lives, we embody what they think we should be without realizing how deeply they affect the person we think we are. And when we find that we are not what we have been told we are, we *reason* what we want to change rather than *embody* the change. Recognizing this subtle difference between reasoning and embodying can help us understand why we are perplexed when we realize that—seemingly inexplicably—we are becoming what we disliked about our parents!

BUILDING A WORTHY SELF

Before we embark on the path to building a worthy self, it's important to clarify the difference between self-worthiness and self-esteem. Although these two terms are often used interchangeably, they are conceptually different. Self-esteem is a concept developed by American psychologists to *measure* self-worthiness. Thus, we can conceive worthiness as the temperature and self-esteem as the thermometer. Another difference is that worthiness is a more stable condition, whereas self-esteem can vary based on context. Although we can feel worthy most of the time, our self-esteem can increase or decrease under certain conditions—increasing, for example, when we receive recognition for an achievement and decreasing when it's ignored by those we choose to love. We increase our worthiness when we embrace the conditions that enhance self-esteem.

In biocognitive theory, self-esteem has three components: *valuation, competence,* and *affiliation.* Each component has conditions that increase or decrease self-esteem. Knowing how to navigate those conditions empowers us to unlearn what has not served us well and to learn the self-worthiness that is our birthright.

Valuation Self-Esteem

The valuation aspect of self-esteem has to do with how much joy we can experience as a result of our positive deeds and fortuitous circumstances. But we must feel valuable before we can appreciate the value of a circumstance. And what governs self-valuation? Self-caring commitments: if you keep self-caring commitments, valuation self-esteem goes up; if you break them, it goes down. After I describe the other two components of self-esteem, I'll explain further.

Competence Self-Esteem

This component of self-esteem identifies how competent we are in what we do professionally and personally: how well we perform at work, at home, in relationships, and with ourselves. If you are learning new ways to improve your relationship with yourself and others, *competence self-esteem* increases. If you stagnate intellectually and emotionally in your professional and personal life, competence self-esteem decreases. If you view change as an opportunity to learn, your competence meter goes up, but if you believe you have little to gain from new learning, it falls.

Affiliation Self-Esteem

This third component of self-esteem has to do with the quality of our relationships and the people we include when we want to share our joy and good fortune. Here we have to be cautious with our selection of coauthors because some may not be willing to celebrate our joy. Fortunately, though, we only need a few good people to achieve healthy affiliation. *Affiliation self-esteem* increases with the quality of people you include in your bioinformational field of joy and celebration, and it decreases with the quantity of people you include who are committed to known misery—theirs and yours.

The biocognitive objective is to increase your self-esteem by establishing a relationship with yourself as if you were your best friend. You can treat yourself as you would treat the friends you most love and admire, in the same ways you would celebrate their good fortunes and protect them from toxic people.

What can make this task difficult is that cultures value collective good more than individual goodness. Self is made a secondary figure in the tribal scheme of things. And in addition to devaluing individuals' attempts to assert their unique selves, tribes support helplessness. A few examples of this should clarify:

* You take yourself to a nice restaurant for a quiet dinner, and the maître d' asks, "Only one?"
* You use a self-caring reason (for example, "I need time to myself") to take a raincheck on an invitation, and you're perceived as being selfish—*but* you will get a pass if you say you're sick or physically unable.
* A friend invites you to a movie and you say, "I would love to go, but I already made plans to meditate this evening." Your friend will most likely respond, "Come on, you can meditate some other time."

Awareness of these implicit tribal biases can help you recognize that you must care for yourself in order to be able to care for others without feeling resentful. But the innate fear of banishment from the tribe can blur your path to abundance, while, paradoxically, genuine self-love leads to the plenitude required to genuinely love others. In chapter 12, you'll learn how you can intentionally build subcultures of wellness that will support you in your self-care.

EMBODYING SELF-WORTHINESS

We progress from the conceptual to the practical understanding that embodiment is one of the most important ingredients in unlearning what does not serve us well and learning the worthiness required to experience abundance without fear. We now know how to work the self-esteem meter to positively affect worthiness—we navigate the realms of value, competence, and affiliation. And we also know the tribal obstacles we may face on our path to self-caring. Our next step is to experientially access the dysfunctional patterns we want to unlearn. Since we learn unwanted patterns of thoughts, emotions, and coauthorship within inseparable fields of bioinformation, the unlearning requires retrieving and experiencing the total mindbody *felt meaning* we are trying to unlearn.

The biocognitive concept of felt meaning is complex and must be patiently unraveled. Some cognitive psychologists propose that when we learn any pattern (functional or dysfunctional), the information is stored as a memory in our brain, and when we recall the experience, it generates thoughts, emotions, and sensations that replicate the experience. This sounds reasonable, and it could persuade us to conclude that we can change any memory, emotion, or action simply by replacing it with another memory, emotion, or action. Fortunately, though, that is not how mindbody change happens, because if it did, you would be no different from your laptop. Computers process data; human beings contextualize meaning.

I trust that you will stay with me as I clarify the concept of felt meaning, because I do not want to dumb down this essential information for fear you cannot understand complex science. Still, before I continue, I must quote what Einstein had to say about stuffy scientists: "If you can't explain it simply, you don't understand it well enough."

So, the simplest way to understand felt meaning is to experience how it surfaces. For example, let's say someone betrayed you when your heart was young. You try to avoid the painful memory, but sometimes it surfaces anyway and ruins your day. You try to convince yourself you can trust again, and you try hard to show that you can. But the moment something goes wrong in a relationship, the ghost of betrayal returns to haunt you. Why can't you simply change what's hurting you so deeply? Are you masochistic? Are you inept? The answer to both questions is an unequivocal *no!* What prevents change is trying to *replace* an unwanted thought pattern with another thought pattern, rather than recontextualizing the felt meaning of the unwanted pattern with the felt meaning of the new pattern you want to *incorporate*. In the example of re-experiencing betrayal, you have done only half the job when those old feelings arise unbidden. You experience the painful memories of the betrayal, but then you attempt to replace the effects of betrayal with wishful thoughts about trusting.

Changing a mindbody experience (an embodied pattern) requires recontextualizing the felt meaning of the experience, not replacing the experience. To recontextualize is to *experience* a new meaning for an old context.

Now would be a good time to take a little break to let these concepts settle before you move ahead to the experiential tools of this chapter.

HOW TO CHANGE THE FELT MEANING OF UNWORTHINESS

Felt meaning is *the experienced significance of a mindbody condition.* If someone tells you they are going to hit you over the head with a bat, you understand the meaning of the threat, but if you are hit with a bat, you experience the felt meaning (pain and shock) of the action. The former is an *image* that has *meaning,* and the latter is an *action* that has *felt meaning.* What would happen if, after you're hit with the bat, you imagine that your head does not hurt anymore? It will not change the painful felt meaning of the hit, nor will any other positive thought or action be able to do so. This example makes the point clearly, but it's easier to understand the pain we feel when we're physically injured than when cultural editors demean us, inflicting emotional pain.

The method I will describe to recontextualize unworthiness works for any of the three components of self-esteem. I suggest you choose the one you think needs most improvement for you at present, but for this exercise I am going to use valuation self-esteem because it is the most important of the three. Feel free to replace my choice with yours if you selected something else.

As in all biocognitive learning experiences, you need to create a state of serenity to quiet your mind and relax your body before you start. Practice the exercise while reading the instructions, until you can do it with your eyes closed. You can use your own relaxation method or one of the contemplative techniques from previous chapters. Regardless of the relaxation method you choose, make the following two commitments as you're slowing down your mind and body:

1 *I am shifting my attention from the outside world to my inside world.* While you're repeating this commitment, check your body for any objections expressed as muscle tension, pain, discomfort, or change in breathing pattern. If any objection emerges, simply observe it without judgment until it passes. If the objection persists, gently shift your attention back and forth from the area affected (the felt meaning of the objection) to an area in your body where there is no objection (the felt meaning of calmness).

2 *I am worth the time I am taking to experience this exercise.* Again, check your body as you make this commitment, and respond to any objection in the same way as you did for the first commitment.

◇◇

Experience Your Felt Meaning of Unworthiness

❖ Recall a situation in which you felt unworthy for something disdainful that you did or that was done to you, an experience of contempt or scorn. Earliest memories are best. Let's say your memory is of being on the playground at school and pulling a little girl's hair. Reenact the negative event visually, including as much detail as you can handle: grabbing a handful of hair, the little girl crying, a teacher running toward you to learn what has happened. After a few minutes of developing the negative experience, as if you were on a theatrical stage, shift from the imagery to the felt meaning the memories bring: instant regret for your action when the girl begins to cry, the fear of punishment. Pay attention to how the felt meaning is manifesting in your body: sensations, discomfort, muscle tension, sadness, or any other negative emotions or unpleasant physical effects.

❖ Pay attention to an area where you sense your inhalations and exhalations (belly, chest, throat, or nose). After a few minutes of focusing on this area, imagine that you can breathe from any part of your body.

❖ Now imagine you're breathing from the area where your felt meaning is expressed as pain, discomfort, change in temperature, or another sensation. Take your time to master this virtual relocation of your breathing. After a few minutes of virtually breathing from the identified felt meaning, shift your attention back to your actual breathing area. Stay grounded in your actual breathing area for a few minutes, and then shift back to the virtual breathing area. If the unworthy felt meaning shifted to a new area of your body, go there and follow the same procedure you used for the previous unworthy felt meaning area.

❖ Continue to shift your focus from the actual breathing area to the virtual breathing area. Notice how your ability to shift from actual to virtual breathing areas improves as you learn this new pattern.

❖ Celebrate with a smile the competence you have gained. Remain relaxed for the next part of the exercise.

◇◇

Experience Your Felt Meaning of Worthiness

❖ Recall a situation when you felt worthy because of something laudable you did or that was done for you. Again, earliest memories are best. Visually reenact the positive circumstance with as much detail as you can recall. For example, you tripped while running down the steps one sunny summer day, and a passing stranger stopped to pick you up, examined your wounds, and stayed with you until you were sure you were okay. After a few minutes of developing the positive experience, as if you were on a theatrical stage, shift from the imagery to the felt meaning the pleasant memories bring. Pay attention to how and where the felt meaning is manifesting in your body: pleasant sensations, joyful emotions, and any other positive physical effects.

❖ Pay attention to the area where you sense your inhalations and exhalations (nose, throat, chest, or belly). After a few minutes of focusing on this breathing area, imagine that you can breathe from any part of your body.

❖ Now imagine you're breathing from the area where your felt meaning is expressed when you recall the worthy circumstances. Take the time to master this virtual relocation of your breathing. After a few minutes of virtually breathing from the identified felt meaning, shift your attention back to your actual breathing area. Stay grounded in your actual breathing area for a few minutes, and then shift back to the virtual breathing area. If the worthy felt meaning shifted to a new place in your body, go there and follow the same procedure you used for the previous felt meaning area. Clear your mindbody by letting your stream of consciousness take you for a ride. Relax.

◇◇◇◇◇◇◇◇◇◇◇◇◇◇◇◇◇◇◇◇◇◇◇◇◇◇◇◇◇◇◇◇◇◇◇◇◇

Recontextualizing Your Felt Meaning of Unworthiness

You have now experienced the felt meanings of unworthiness and worthiness, a powerful tool in working with the mindbody code. Each of these felt meanings has its own characteristics and areas of manifestation. The next few steps are the most important.

❖ Visually recall an unworthy memory and identify where its felt meaning surfaces. Now release your attention from the imagery and experience the area where the felt meaning emerged. Stay with the discomfort it may trigger for a few minutes. Don't forget to breathe!

❖ Visually recall a worthy memory and identify where its felt meaning surfaces. Then release the imagery and experience the area where the felt meaning appeared. For a few minutes, stay with the comfort it may trigger. Breathe.

❖ Finally, shift from the felt meaning of unworthiness to the felt meaning of worthiness as you experience it in your body. Stay with each condition for about a minute before shifting to the other condition. Continue the shifting for no longer than four to five minutes.

❖ Notice the felt meaning of unworthiness beginning to weaken and dissipate. If this does not happen right away, don't worry. It just needs a bit more work another day.

❖ Count slowly from one to five and open your eyes. Before you get up, gently look around until you feel reoriented.

❖ ❖ ❖

You have taken a significant step in biocognitive learning in this chapter; you have experienced working in your internal world to recontextualize unworthy felt meaning with worthy felt meaning. But since the neuro-maps of your beliefs require new evidence in order to increase or decrease the strength of their connections, you need to create additional evidence that supports worthiness consciousness. In other words, you have shaken up your belief horizons and cracked your ceilings of abundance. Now you need to increase your capacity for self-caring, commit to new learn-ing, and take an honest look at the quality of your present coauthors. If you continue to work on the three components of self-esteem I intro-duced you to in this chapter and invest your time and energy in people who will gladly coauthor your worthiness, your fear of abundance will recontextualize. It will transform into living with joy as your birthright.

In the next chapter, I will introduce you to a fascinating manifesta-tion of the mindbody code that offers further insights into wounds and healing: the physical phenomenon of stigmata.

Stigmata:
How the Mind Wounds
and Heals the Body

I n this chapter, I'll share what I've learned from my investigations with
stigmatics and how their extraordinary beliefs helped me understand
the mindbody code. Stigmatics are people who develop physical wounds
that resemble those of Christ, with no attributable physical cause. Let's
examine this question: what are the conditions necessary for the mind to
wound the body in this way—or to heal it?

Saint Francis of Assisi received the stigmata (the wounds of Christ) in
1224 AD, after fasting for forty days on La Verna. Although it was the first
recorded account of this mysterious phenomenon, some scholars suggest
that Saint Paul's words—"I bear in my body the marks of the Lord Jesus"
(Galatians 6:17)—may qualify him as the first stigmatic, if his statement
is taken literally. Two years before the Saint Francis incident, a monk in
Oxford claimed to be the redeemer of mankind and proclaimed that his
five crucifixion wounds were the work of God. After being arrested for
blasphemy, however, he confessed they were self-inflicted. Some speculate
torture was engaged to persuade him to confess. Since the time of Saint
Francis, almost four hundred cases of stigmata have been recorded.

The Vatican's position continues to be that the question of whether
stigmata are the result of divine intervention or are self-initiated is up to

each individual's belief. And since the time of the apostles, the Vatican has not recognized divine intervention.

My interest in stigmata is biocognitive rather than theological. There is substantial evidence in scientific literature that indicates our thoughts and beliefs affect our immune system and ultimately our health. Observing acts of compassion can increase antibodies that fight upper respiratory infections. Placebos (expectations of healing) can have the same pain-relieving effects as narcotics. Nocebo (expectation of harm) injections can constrict or dilate the bronchial airways, depending on the expectation presented to the subject—despite the injections being nothing more than saline water. Confession decreases blood pressure, heart rate, and stress hormones such as cortisol while increasing immune function.

So if we exclude divine intervention and self-infliction, what can be said about these crucifixion-like wounds in light of evidence that they resist infection and that the affected do not develop anemia despite daily loss of blood? Padre Pio, who was canonized in 2002, not for his stigmata but for his devotional deeds, is said to have bled a cup of blood a day for nearly fifty years without deleterious effects.

But before discussing the psychology (or, I should say, the biocognition) of stigmata, let me bring up another perplexing characteristic that merits consideration. Medieval artists depicted Christ on the cross with wounds on the palm of his hands. Forensic scientists suggest the Romans knew that if the palms were nailed, they would not be able to sustain the weight of the body, so they nailed the wrists instead. The Shroud of Turin and other evidence confirms the forensic findings.

There is no more compelling evidence that our biology conforms to our beliefs than the fact that before the scientific evidence about the anatomy of crucifixion was available, stigmatics manifested their wounds on their palms, while in contemporary cases, the wounds appear on the wrists. Also of interest is that attempts to produce the wounds under hypnosis have failed.

Given what I've shared so far, then, what is the mindbody process of stigmata? I suggest that in order to begin to understand the motivational components of stigmata, we need to examine the medieval Christian model of suffering.

In those days, suffering was considered the way to identify with Christ. The tormented lives of the Catholic mystics of that era provide ample evidence to support this penance model. So if suffering was the way to identify with Christ, to replicate his wounds would certainly be the ultimate achievement. The personal accounts of some stigmatics praying for their wounds support the contention that suffering was a desired state.

The apparent power of the mindbody process to manifest suffering in the flesh could have significant implications. Consider this: if belief can injure tissue by identifying with the suffering of Christ, identifying with the love of Christ could have powerful healing effects for Catholic cultures. And I emphasize Catholics because 99 percent of stigmatics are Catholic; beliefs gain power when shared within a culture. If stigmatics can potentially bypass the harmful physical consequences of their wounds by creating a unique immune condition, we can only imagine what we could achieve if we learned the biocognition of love.

Science has advanced to a level where the consequences of prayer, faith, and love can be measured and harnessed to accomplish healing rather than promote suffering. Research is presently under way to study changes in the molecular structure of water that has been blessed, the effects of compassionate imagery on the growth rate of malignant cells, and the role of faith in spontaneous healing.

IDENTIFYING WOUNDING AND HEALING CONTEXTS

Every condition has its opposite, and beliefs that can wound are no exception. Although cases of stigmata are extremely rare, they share contributing factors with the nocebo effect reported frequently in medical literature. You are told you have an illness, which, based on the average mortality for that illness, means you have six months to live. But rather than hearing the word "average" you hear *how long* you are expected to live. In fact, you are usually given the dire news without the "specialist" mentioning that this "sentencing" is based on an average rather than an absolute. I consider this approach both predatory and unscientific.

Let's examine the dynamics of this type of medical "sentencing." A nocebo effect is triggered by a cultural editor (doctor) with corroborating evidence that, on the average, patients with your diagnosis die within the prognosticated time. You have an authority pontificating with evidence. How can you argue with that? Let's do it by battling the science of averages with the science of individual differences. In this example, although the average life expectancy is six months, the left side of a chart of the normal distribution for this illness may be five weeks and the right may be eight years. The strongest nocebo effect lies around the left end and the strongest placebo effect around the right end. But unfortunately, conventional researchers consider both extremes of the distribution "nuisance variables" to be discarded. This scientific myopia robs patients of the most powerful mindbody weapon responsible for spontaneous remission, unexpected recovery, and survival of mistaken diagnosis: the power of belief that can trigger a *healing response.*

We all have a healing response, but most of us need permission from a cultural authority or deity to activate our power to overcome the averages. Stigmatics present a category that has not been studied in academic biology: wounding based on divine belief. In other words, placebo heals and nocebo harms—but stigmata is a *revered* wound. How can this rare condition enhance our understanding of how the mindbody code works? Although stigmatics experience their pain as if their hands/wrists and feet were pierced with crucifixion nails, they do not take pain medication or lose consciousness. There is much scientific evidence showing that the perception of pain is strongly influenced by cultural contexts. For example, if you fracture your leg falling down a set of stairs that are badly maintained by your negligent landlord, you will feel significantly more pain than if you were to fracture it by diving off a cliff to save a drowning child.

Beliefs can wound, heal, and interpret pain based on cultural contexts. Our environment, genetics, and cultural editors are coauthors of our health and illness. But are we able to change those beliefs that no longer serve us well? We can certainly change any belief if we are willing to look beyond the pale.

SPONTANEOUS HEALING AROUND STIGMATICS

Conventional science is unable to explain spontaneous healing: the immediate transformation from illness to health. Health professionals call it spontaneous remission, religions call it miracle, and shamans call it magic. But independent of the label given, spontaneous healing occurs much more frequently than is reported in scientific literature. This is because it takes place at the edge of the curve or normal distribution, so it is discarded as a nuisance variable—a topic not worthy of publication.

Yet spontaneous healing is not uncommon among Catholics who come into contact with stigmatics. Sharing the psychospiritual culture of Catholicism permits the possibility of healing because in that culture, stigmata are considered divine. But to best explain the dynamics of spontaneous healing, I will share an investigation I conducted for National Geographic.

The stigmatic was a woman in Mexico City who exhibited a deep wound on her forehead in the shape of a cross. In the past, she had also produced wounds on her wrists and feet, but these had healed at the time I saw her. This particular investigation was significant because it was the first time in the history of stigmatics that anyone had conducted immunological studies. By considering the phenomenon from this perspective, we were able to see how her biology was responding to her stigmata. Because of the depth of her wound, her intense pain, her level of stress related to her fear of being filmed, the continuous bleeding, and the lack of infection, we were expecting something very different from what we found.

First, the depth of the wound indicated it was highly unlikely that it had been self-inflicted: an intentional deep cut in the form of a cross would tear tissue irregularly at the junction of the vertical and horizontal lines, and we did not find this. Other laboratory tests confirmed that the wound had torn deep tissue. We expected to see high levels of antibodies and pro-inflammatory secretion resulting from an effort to protect and repair the wound, a high level of cortisol indicating stress, and heightened levels of red blood cells compensating for the frequent bleeding. To our immense surprise, when we ran tests to gauge these factors, all her lab results were within normal limits. There was no anemia, no infection, and no healing of the open wound—without any help from her immune system!

These results were astonishing enough, but the most remarkable finding was that two spontaneous healings took place around this stigmatic woman. A boy with leukemia and a man with prostate cancer had both gone into remission. When I interviewed the physician who had examined the stigmatic as well as the two spontaneously healed patients, her response was telling: "In medical school, we are not trained to understand these conditions. I simply call it a miracle."

THE ATONEMENT ARCHETYPE

Based on extensive research into other cultures and religions, I propose that feeling a need to suffer is not a condition limited to Catholics. Although it may take different forms, most cultures and their religions share a universal condition I call the atonement archetype. One must suffer either before reaching desired goals or because of past conduct. It seems to me that Western cultures subscribe to the premise of suffering for future gains, whereas Eastern cultures suffer from past karmic deeds. Of course, there are those who are so guilt-ridden that they subscribe to both modes of suffering. But the relevance here in examining our own suffering is that many of us carry our own version of stigmata: a stigma unrelated to the wounds of Christ's crucifixion. This need to suffer has a powerful detrimental effect on our wellness and contributes to our illnesses.

Clearly, in the process of living we are confronted with challenges and misfortunes that cause some of our suffering and are beyond our control. By contrast, what I am addressing here is the cultural beliefs that *welcome* our external conditions of suffering and create our own internal hell—not because life itself can be painful but because we deserve to suffer as a way to atone for our misdeeds. Given these powerful tribal beliefs, are we doomed to suffer? No, but we must go beyond the pale if we want alternatives to the atonement archetype. What we learn within the pale can best be unlearned outside of it. Although I've previously mentioned the biocognitive concept of the tribal pale, its application here is to achieve freedom from *learned suffering*. Yes, most suffering is learned!

We are not born with a need to atone by suffering for our misdeeds. We coauthor this need with our cultural and spiritual leaders within the tribal pale. But before we delve deeper, I want to be clear that I am not suggesting we should dismiss our wrongdoing without consequences.

Instead, we can take responsibility for our misdeeds by taking corrective action rather than atoning for them by suffering. In fact, punishment does little to change behavior—it simply suppresses it.

For a closer look at learned suffering and its power to heal and wound, let's return to the stigmatic woman I investigated. She traveled throughout Mexico to share her stigmata experience, and during her journey, a few people around her also had spontaneous healings, as I mentioned. It was even said that merely seeing her and her wound during a television interview was sufficient to trigger spontaneous healings in some believers.

I inserted myself into the stigmata experience by teaching her a way to reduce the excruciating pain she experienced by 80 percent, using a method of identifying with love rather than suffering—and the sign of the cross on her forehead healed within a few weeks. And here is the amazing consequence: when I interviewed her again a year later, she told me the wound on her forehead had returned. She explained to me that when she shared her story without the wound, the spontaneous healings stopped. She had concluded that without the wound, she could have no healing effect on others. She further reasoned that, since the level of pain she experienced remained at only 20 percent of its former strength, she could live with it if it would continue to trigger spontaneous healings. The cross on her forehead did not heal again.

This was a lesson of learned suffering within the pale: she had to suffer or healing could not occur.

I will admit that my first reaction upon hearing this was to suspect she had inflicted the wound herself in order to help others. But when I spoke to her doctor again, she reported witnessing the wound's reappearance on her patient's forehead. Small red dots began to appear in a vertical line, followed by a horizontal one, and the two lines slowly intersected to depict a perfect cross. Then, gradually, the wound deepened and formed a thick scab that bled irregularly.

What can we conclude from this extraordinary sequence of events? Independent of whether the gash was self-inflicted, let's look at the beliefs that led to the results.

The stigmatic: The woman believed the wound was necessary for spontaneous healings to take place; a need to demonstrate suffering was fundamental. Additionally, she believed that her suffering was a gift, given to her in order to heal others. This signaled her biology to both suspend healing and prevent infection of the wound.

The spontaneously healed: The belief that the wound was an act of divine intervention triggered their spontaneous healing. Through it, they found *permission* to activate their own healing response.

Under these circumstances, shared beliefs within the pale had a beneficial effect.

What is significant here is that coauthored beliefs can wound and heal the body in ways that conventional biology cannot explain. This is not because a cogent explanation is impossible but because reductionist biology does not explain what it cannot measure within its model of physical cause and effect. Still, we don't have to go to the other extreme and be satisfied with esoteric explanations. In chapter 3, I offered scientific evidence of how thoughts and emotions can influence nervous, immune, and endocrine regulation. In biocognition, I incorporate this mindbody evidence, along with research into how cultures affect brain function, to argue that symbols become biosymbols as they are assimilated by our culturally influenced perception. What we believe is more than our thoughts; it is embodied biology in culturally defined contexts.

My objective here is to argue the power of cultural beliefs in the healing and wounding processes and leave the spiritual interpretation of these phenomena to theologians. We can learn from extraordinary experiences and apply their beneficial effects to more commonplace conditions. But to do this, we must be willing to accept that our mindbody can achieve much more than what our scientific instruments can record and measure.

LEARNING HOW TO GET SICK

Illness is a clever condition we learn in order to distract ourselves from either an overwhelming impasse or from sustainable joy. Genetic predispositions wait patiently to be triggered into either disharmony or wellness—a choice of self-devaluation or self-worthiness. Of course, a prolonged "illness" can reach a critical physical mass, making it irreversible. At that level, only a metabiological shift of mindbody consciousness can reverse what conventional medicine calls "terminal illness." It is essential to understand, however, that you must never blame yourself or be persuaded to accept blame for an illness. There are conditions in which a higher order of consciousness decides it's time to release the body and move on to another dimension. But meanwhile, you can learn the biocognition of love to slowly relinquish your atonement archetype. I say *slowly* because the felt meaning of a belief requires time to recontextualize the mindbody learning that produced the dysfunctional condition you want to change.

For example, medical intervention (biochemical or surgical) only treats the critical mass created by the illness, without addressing the causes of health we neglected when we learned the illness. In other words, reductionist medicine may be necessary, but it is not sufficient for sustainable healing.

As you develop a dysfunctional behavior, you teach *all* your mindbody to get sick. For example, if you live in a chronic state of anger because you believe the world is unfair to you—whether this is true or not—this belief teaches your nervous system to remain on chronic hyperalarm, your immune system to underrespond to pathogens and to secrete molecules that cause inflammation, and your endocrine system to increase stress hormones that damage tissue. What did your belief teach your mindbody? Possibly cardiovascular disease, cerebral vascular disease, or other learned diseases. It does not mean, however, that anger causes these diseases. Instead, chronic anger (out of context) is what causes the damage that eventually surfaces as disease. In fact, anger appropriate to a circumstance is actually good for your immune system! For example, if someone betrays you, anger is an appropriate emotion that helps you emerge from the disillusionment you feel, but if you continue to be angry in the face of loyalty, you turn a righteous emotion into a toxic expression.

LOVE AS ANTIDOTE TO YOUR LEARNED SUFFERING

I hope that learning the dynamics of stigmata has helped you see the power of belief in the processes of healing and wounding. What is important to take away from this lesson is that the power lies in the belief, whether that belief is true or not. Similarly, my work with centenarians has shown me that their belief that most people love them, whether accurate or not, is one of the main contributors to their longevity. But rather than assuming you can change your beliefs by simply reasoning it's good for you to do so, I propose you learn sufficient self-worthiness to accept the benefits of your new belief.

Paradoxically, stigmatics accept their suffering as a gift of divine love. Does this mean that they lack self-worthiness and that love requires suffering? The answers illustrate that love, self-worthiness, and suffering require untangling before you can recontextualize learned suffering. Stigmatics relinquish their worthiness because of their love for God. In fact, they believe they are *not worthy* to receive the divine gift of suffering. This belief shows how love can be misguided when suffering is perceived as a necessary condition. More important, relinquishing self-worthiness in the name of love precludes self-love; it negates a necessary condition to recontextualize learned suffering.

Applying the extraordinary dynamics of stigmata to more ordinary painful circumstances will help you understand why people in abusive relationships perceive the abuse as an expression of love from the abuser. Without disrespect for the religious beliefs of stigmatics and their followers, I argue that when we relinquish our self-worthiness to others, we entangle love with suffering. Thus, the self-worthiness I propose here is founded on self-love: the entanglement with suffering decreases as self-love increases.

But how can you differentiate self-worthiness from narcissistic love? The distinction is that narcissists develop an exaggerated sense of personal value to compensate for their perceived unworthiness. They try hard to make others believe what they profoundly doubt in themselves. In contrast, authentic self-worth is your capacity to accept love from yourself and offer it to others, based on your own dignity and compassion. The dignity and compassion I am referring to come from personal experience, not wishful thinking.

BREAKING THE POTENTIAL CIRCULARITY OF LOVE

A vague description of love can lead to a circular definition and misuse of its power; possessing the self-worthiness necessary to accept love, and love being based on dignity and compassion may seem circular. In other words, if your capacity to accept love defines your self-worthiness, if you don't already feel self-worthy, how can you accept love? And if loving yourself and others comes from your own sense of dignity and compassion, how can you have dignity and compassion if you lack self-love? See the circularity? I am not trying to confuse you, so let me explain. Self-evidence is your key to avoiding the potential circularity of love.

Imagine that you are building a tower of love. The builder is your own self-worth, and the materials you are using to build love are your dignity and compassion. The builder (self-worth) has built other towers (you have loved before) and knows from past experience how to use the materials (you have acted with dignity and compassion before). The builder cannot construct the tower without having experience; you gain it as you perfect your craft. In other words, unless you have lived from birth in an isolated cave, you already have the dignity and compassion you need in order to feel worthy of accepting love. It is a matter of accessing the memories that contain the felt meaning of your worthy deeds. They're all there, but inaccessible, when you avoid loving yourself.

TURNING KNOWLEDGE INTO HEALING TOOLS

Now let's apply practical tools to what you have learned in this chapter. Let me remind you, these methods are not reasoning processes; they are based on powerful mindbody code principles that work indirectly and subtly to yield lasting change.

◇◇◇

Unlearning Self-Imposed Suffering

❖ Identify your tribal and religious authorities to find the model of suffering you were taught. For example, suffering to reach success, wealth, wisdom, or heaven.

❖ Observe what you feel in your mindbody when you discover how you were taught suffering. Was it a religious authority, a book, a teacher, a parent?

❖ Who continues to remind you that you should suffer? Are the cultural editors still in your life, or people who have passed on, or who live nearby or far from you?

❖ Recall a significant circumstance in which you learned suffering and identify the coauthors and context. For example, you went away to college against your parents' wishes, and were reminded you had made an "unwise" decision every time you came home for summer breaks. Allow the mindbody expression of the memory to unfold. *Do not blame—simply observe.*

❖ Commit to recalling how you were taught to suffer the next time you fall into a suffering mode. We fall into default modes from past experiences. For example, the suffering response is triggered by learned associations with coauthors and dysfunctional circumstances.

❖ Any time you enter learned suffering, recall a memory of dignity and compassion. For example, when you graduated from college, you thanked your parents for loving you, without making them feel guilty for not supporting your decision. Shift from the mindbody experience of suffering to the dignity and compassion experience and observe without expectations. Your mindbody code trumps suffering with the felt meaning of dignity and compassion. It works in very subtle and indirect ways.

Freedom from Your Atonement Archetype

How do you punish yourself when you do something wrong? Do you sabotage your joy, overeat, abuse drugs, gamble, engage in promiscuous sex, or find other ways of paying for your bad deeds?

❖ Recall a recent situation in which you used the type of punishment you identified. Where and how do you experience the memory in your mindbody? Observe without judging.

❖ Do you believe you have to pay for your sins? If you do, where did you learn this? Is it affecting your health, wealth, or love?

❖ Identify what area in your life is negatively affected. For example, if it's your health, is there a pattern of getting sick? If it's wealth, is there a pattern of losing or not making enough money? If it's love, what is the pattern of conflict in your relationships?

❖ Consider that rather than paying for your bad deeds or "sins" with suffering, you can take corrective action. Identify what your mindbody feels when you imagine an alternative response to suffering as punishment.

❖ What alternative action did you choose to replace learned suffering? The corrective action must include self-compassion and dignity. What does your mindbody feel when you consider your new alternatives? Simply observe.

❖ Commit to applying your new corrective action next time you determine you have to atone for a bad deed. What authority must you defy if you give up your atonement model of suffering? Without interpretation, observe how you experience defying this authority in your mindbody.

◇◇◇◇◇◇◇◇◇◇◇◇◇◇◇◇◇◇◇◇◇◇◇◇◇◇◇◇

Unlearning Illness

Please note: these methods should be used in conjunction with professional medical assistance, not as a replacement for it.

* Identify a dysfunction or illness you may have. Do not set expectations of healing, improving, or worsening. For example, if you have diabetes, rather than set healing goals, learn what causes of health you are neglecting by teaching your mindbody conditions that worsen your illness. Healing is achieved with indirect actions. You did not learn an illness intellectually. It is a dysfunctional mindbody process that requires more than reasoning.

* Identify people and contexts that increase or decrease your symptoms or need for medication. This instruction does not mean you should self-medicate or change your medication without consulting your health care professional.

* Identify what or who makes your symptoms increase and decrease. How are you responding and feeling in each circumstance? What differences do you notice?

* Associate decreased symptoms with conditions of empowerment and increased symptoms with conditions of helplessness. Who taught you each of the conditions, and which do you express more frequently in your daily activities? Empowerment

means accessing the resources you need to overcome a challenge. Helplessness means having no access to resources or not seeking them when they are available.

❖ After identifying empowering behaviors and conditions, gradually incorporate them into your daily activities. For example, if you are often depressed, you can decide to exercise instead of investing in self-pity. As you increase empowerment mindfulness, you will be able to decrease helplessness more effectively.

❖ When you notice improvements, remember that there is more to do. Your new empowerment mindfulness is still fragile and requires practice. Even so, unlearning bad patterns takes less time than learning them.

❖ How does your felt meaning of empowerment manifest in your mindbody? For example, what do you experience when you access new resources to overcome old challenges?

❖ Find people and contexts that enhance your new empowering initiative and celebrate with them. Celebrations do not need to be elaborate. A simple expression of gratitude is more than sufficient.

❖ Now identify people and contexts that make it difficult for you to improve your condition—for example, someone who is also often depressed and wants to coauthor misery. Do they remind you that you are not worthy of your improvements? Are they your coauthors of illness? Remember, coauthors are usually not aware of their negative contributions, and some are not willing to accept feedback from you.

❖ Limit your contact with coauthors of illness—for example, people who remind you of your condition and identify you with your condition. Evaluate whether it's worth it for you to continue seeing them. If it is, limit your contact and focus on the quality rather than the quantity of time you spend together.

❖ ❖ ❖

As with all the practical applications I present at the end of each chapter, these should be incorporated gradually, as mindful rituals in your life, to replace the mindless habits that obstruct your wellness. You can also review any of the chapters at any time to reinforce what you learned there and apply it to your life.

Forgiveness as Liberation from Self-Entrapment

A few years ago I gave a lecture at Galway Cathedral in Ireland titled "The Psychology of Forgiveness: Liberation from Self-Entrapment." The cathedral was packed with people hungry for this information. After I finished, a priest came up to me at the podium and said, "I am so pleased you presented this lecture because, as priests, we tell our parishioners to forgive, but we don't teach them how to do it." Then a man leaning heavily on crutches came slowly toward me and said, "I have a debilitating autoimmune disease. Do you think there is still hope for me?"

The priest confirmed that I was teaching something direly needed, and the man on crutches made me wonder if losing hope and holding grudges are a prescription for disease. After many years of teaching and refining biocognitive methods that enable people to forgive at the deepest mindbody level, I can tell you that most cultural and spiritual editors continue to instill the value of forgiveness without providing any effective tools for doing so. Similarly, although many health care professionals warn that holding grudges causes debilitating stress that can lead to illness, they fail to understand that self-entrapment is the real culprit. They address the effect without recognizing the cause.

In this chapter, I'll teach you a mindbody process that releases blocks to forgiveness and illustrates, experientially, how reluctance to forgive is a form of self-entrapment that negatively affects your health and longevity. I'll also show you why resolving forgiveness intellectually is not sufficient to achieve mindbody liberation from the enslavement that holding grudges creates. Interestingly, forgiveness has little to do with the perpetrator who has committed a harmful act against us and much to do with the experience of disempowerment that follows.

When we are physically or emotionally assaulted, we respond with the primitive part of our brain that is designed to react without intellectual processing. It responds with reflexes, not logic. Any threatening situation requires instantaneous action, leaving the interpretation of what has taken place for the more complex part of the brain. (Reasoning comes after the danger has passed.) Knowing this survival mechanism will help you understand why forgiving an assault upon your worthiness requires more than reasoning. In fact, if you rely on reasoning to forgive a painful misdeed, you will access only how you interpreted the misdeed, not what actually happened to you.

A PATH TO FORGIVENESS

If forgiving were merely an intellectual endeavor, you would only need to convince yourself there was a good reason to do it: that forgiving is humane, compassionate, good for your health, valued by society and religion, and so on. That's what most people do, thinking the triggering event is behind them. But unfortunately, whenever they think about the person or situation they thought they had forgiven, they still find anger, sadness, and resentment surfacing to remind them their wound remains unhealed. Why do I insist that forgiveness requires more than reasoning? The answer is complex, which is why I dedicate an entire chapter to helping you understand and successfully resolve the challenges that block your forgiveness. But before you look into how to forgive, you need to understand the nature of what you want to forgive and how a wound is inflicted when wrongful action is perpetrated against you.

Helplessness

Forgiving involves empowerment because the misdeed perpetrated against you renders you helpless. If you don't regain the empowerment you relinquished to your perpetrator, you cannot reach a state of forgiveness. Another way of looking at this is that *you gave away* what you thought *someone else took* from you. At the time of the misdeed, you were not aware of giving the perpetrator permission to rob you of your worthiness. Although I am using reasoning to explain the dynamics of a misdeed, toward the end of the chapter I'll teach you how to embody each intellectual part of the lesson and experientially regain your empowerment. (You first learn the rules of the game, and then you play it.)

The Wounds

Self-worthiness is the value you assign to your identity based on your personal accomplishments and feedback from your cultural editors. *Empowerment* is the capacity to access resources when confronted with a challenge. Archetypal wounds diminish both self-worthiness and empowerment. If you lack or are denied needed resources, you feel helpless.

When you're wounded, especially by significant people in your life, your empowerment is challenged, and your worthiness is called into question. The vulnerability your loss of empowerment creates within you allows the wound to damage your worthiness. Just as a protective vest can keep a gunshot from wounding you, a sense of worthiness protects you from the wounds of others' misdeeds, or at least minimizes the damage.

Your interpretation of your wound is subjectively based on your cultural history of shame, abandonment, or betrayal. Given the nature of these three archetypal wounds, the interpretation you make of the misdeed determines the healing field you need to access to resolve it. This is another important component of forgiveness; before you can forgive at the deepest level, you must apply the proper antidote to heal your wound. Before this chapter comes to a close, I will show you how to identify and apply the proper healing field.

RELINQUISHING VICTIMHOOD

Since misdeeds disempower us, we devise clever, albeit dysfunctional, ways to compensate for our loss. We find power in victimhood and remain there until we are willing and able to forgive. Sadly, the tribes in which we live support such victimhood in very interesting ways. If you are unjustly wronged, the tribe usually offers sympathy and recognition that this happened. This is not what you need; you need a path to liberation. Relinquishing victimhood requires regaining your worthiness and finding alternatives to these poor substitutes for forgiveness.

For example, let's say your partner betrays you, and the tribe finds out, either through gossip or because your need for empathy drives you to disclose the betrayal. Though you need empathy to reconfirm your worthiness, you find only tribal sympathy that keeps you trapped in victimhood. Paradoxically, the healthy validation you seek in the tribe is inadvertently given in a way that further invalidates you. Why? There are many reasons, but I will offer you the most relevant to mindbody forgiveness.

Whereas empathy empowers you by affirming your tribal worthiness, sympathy offers only pity for your helplessness. The former reminds you of your strength, and the latter confirms your weakness. Tribes support helplessness within the pale, and discourage empowerment beyond the pale. Why? Because when you succeed beyond the pale, you no longer need the tribe; the tribe insists upon dependence at any expense.

THE BIOCOGNITIVE SPACE OF THE PERPETRATOR

When we perceive the world around us, we impose our cultural history on our perception. The world is open to your coauthoring of the biocognitive space you choose. For example, flowers could remind you of your first love or your first visit to a funeral home. Your biocognitive space of *flowers* is contextualized based on your cultural history rather than some static construction that everyone perceives equally. Interestingly, the color white has the connotation of purity in most Western cultures, and is associated with death in some Eastern cultures. Thus, we view the world based on what we *culturally* learn to see. Now you will *see* how this brief lesson in cultural neuroscience can help you understand the biocognitive space you create of a perpetrator whom you have been reluctant or unable to forgive.

Accepting that you are the coauthor of your biocognitive space will allow you to own your part in the formulation of the wound and the role you have assigned the one who perpetrated it upon you. But owning coauthorship does not mean you should blame yourself for the misdeed committed against you. Instead, I will show you how misdeeds are structured intellectually. And toward the end of the chapter, I'll teach you how to experientially find freedom from self-entrapment through embodied forgiveness: mindbody recontextualizing of the misdeed, the chosen wound, and the interpreted space you give the perpetrator.

How We Choose Our Wounds

We choose our wounds? I realize this notion may seem strange at first, as might the idea that we choose how we interpret the misdeeds perpetrated against us. But I don't mean we make these choices because we are simpleminded or masochistic. Instead, because we are complex sentient beings, we trust others to behave with dignity and compassion. Trust entails being vulnerable enough to be deceived and disappointed. And the unique vulnerability that identifies your humanity is what permits you to categorize your wounds.

You are more susceptible to holding grudges if your cultural editors wounded you early on in your personal journey. Why? Because, since insults to your worthiness make you more vulnerable to later wounds, you learn to replace your lost worthiness with victimhood—at the encouragement of your tribe. The wound you choose in order to interpret your pain becomes a shield of protection against forgiving because releasing your grudge means being vulnerable again. Yes, it is a perplexing process, so let's use an example to clarify.

Suppose your mother shames you in front of your best friend when you are nine years old. Perhaps she tells you to stop eating the pizza you and your friend are enjoying because she has noticed you're getting fat. You are deeply hurt, and you resent your mother for saying such a thing in front of your friend and ruining your fun. Time passes, and you forget the incident until, fifteen years later, you feel the same pain, with greater intensity, when your partner shames you at a party, making a similar comment. Unforgiven grudges have a cumulative effect. Each of these wounds adds to your unresolved helplessness, but instead of confronting the reason you feel helpless, you embrace your grudge with greater determination to fight back: a rebel with a mistaken cause.

Also, since shame was the archetypal wound that your significant cultural editor (mother) inflicted upon you, you are more likely to choose shame when you interpret insults to your worthiness in the future. Recall that when we are wounded early in life by people we love, they teach us to entangle love with our wound.

At some point in your life, your grudge becomes an unwelcome burden, you realize you have to let go, and you attempt to "forgive." But since you do not understand the complexity of mindbody wounding, you intellectually conclude that you can release your grudge simply by reasoning that it's the right thing to do. You feel some relief from this, and you assume the conflict is resolved—until the resentment comes back to haunt you when you think about the transgression again. Unfortunately, when this happens, you are likely to blame yourself for your failure to do the "right thing" by forgiving, and you take another hit to your worthiness.

This vicious cycle of emotional helplessness is not caused by a flaw in your character. It is the result of not yet knowing an effective path to resolution. It is vital that you grasp this distinction so you may begin your process of forgiveness as self-liberation.

It's also important to understand that this is a *process* rather than a technique. A technique is a useful tool for solving a specific problem, but a process, as I define it in biocognition, is a path to changing a way of life. You forgive to free yourself from the enslavement of past grudges and fortify yourself against future wounds by drawing on your worthiness rather than victimhood.

In working with siblings who were abused by the same parent, I've found that the misdeed is interpreted subjectively by each child. For example, two daughters were sexually abused by their father but one *chose* shame, and the other betrayal, to interpret the same wound. As you may recall from chapter 2, shame is experienced as humiliation, and betrayal as a violation of trust. Both are dreadful, but each is conceptualized with an individuality that cannot be compromised by any amount of abuse. This highly subjective process of choosing your archetypal wound illustrates the importance of identifying the type of wound behind your grudge, before you attempt to forgive. If you do not take this essential step, it's like prescribing medication without first correctly diagnosing the illness.

THE LOSS OF INNOCENCE

Being wounded challenges our expectations of what is best in others. We assume most people are kind, considerate, fair, and sensitive. Thus when we are shamed, betrayed, or abandoned for the first time, our pristine concept of humanity is badly shaken. And the turbulence is most intense when we are wounded by a cultural editor we love. Not only do we question our assumptions of relationships, but, more important, we also question the essence of love itself.

Of course, you don't do any of this analysis consciously or deliberately, but it leaves an imprint of doubt at the deepest level of your identity. If you are wounded before you're old enough to abstract information, you blame *all* of yourself, but if you are older, you only blame your conduct. For example, if you're wounded at six years of age, you conclude you are a bad *person,* but if it happens when you're fifteen, you blame what you *did* as the cause of wounding. Later, as you learn to differentiate further, the act of blaming yourself transitions to resenting the person who wounded you. You move from self-deprecation to constructing a grudge.

This process shows how we interpret misdeeds based on our developmental stage, but it also illustrates how we fail to see what has actually been damaged. We can blame all of what we are, part of what are, or the perpetrator, without recognizing that the wound is at heart a powerful blow to our worthiness. *Lacking awareness of what was truly damaged within us,* we hopelessly miss the mark when we try to forgive. To comply with cultural expectations, we focus on the grudge and the redemption of the perpetrator rather than on identifying that our real wound is that we have lost a sense of our own worthiness—a necessary understanding to liberate ourselves from self-entrapment.

Perhaps now you can begin to appreciate that forgiveness is one of the most complex acts of self-love you will encounter on your personal journey. The difficulty lies in not understanding the comprehensiveness of what you want to forgive. Many failures in life have to do with trying to solve experiential problems with intellectualized solutions. Intellect is necessary to conceptualize our working strategies, but we get lost when we assume that thoughts can embrace experience.

RECONCILIATION AND REDEMPTION

In the process of forgiving, reconciling with the perpetrator is only an option, not a necessity. Some people are reluctant to forgive because they think they will have to "make up" with the person who wounded them, but this is not so. Another misconception that blocks forgiving is the belief that if you do reconcile, you must redeem the perpetrator. But consider this: it would be next to impossible to reconcile with and see as redeemed someone who killed your child! The forgiveness process I'll teach you will liberate you without your having to reconcile with or redeem those who have inflicted pain. How is that possible? Let me give you an intellectual conceptualization before offering the experiential resolution.

Since we conceptualize the perpetrator within our biocognitive space based on our cultural interpretation of what has taken place, we choose the wound, the grudge, and the requirements for forgiveness. But this is a culturally constructed scenario rather than an absolute. Can the director of a play change the script? Imagine your culture as the playwright, and you are the director of your play. The culture sets the parameters, and you interpret your world within them. If you ask the playwright to change the script, your request will most likely be denied. But what if you could conceive the play differently? You could create your own *adaptation* of the play. And that is precisely what you do with the biocognitive process of forgiveness.

Adapting New Scripts from Old Tribal Plays

Continuing to apply the theater metaphor, you can explore how to change the cultural play of forgiveness your cultural editors have written for you. The new script is based on recovering your empowerment and self-worth, releasing your grudge, and healing your archetypal wound.

As the director of an adaptation, you can relinquish victimhood with all its tribal benefits—the old play. You can replace the coauthors of the original script with characters who are willing to support your new script of forgiveness. And you can acknowledge the playwright's original contribution without having to suffer its limitations. Although your cultural editors write the play, you, as director of your personal journey, adapt it to fit your need to grow and transcend. Just remember, your audience may not like your adaptation. You will have conceived the new script beyond the pale and without permission from the playwright. This means you may have to find a new audience that can appreciate the worthiness of your adaptation. But you are the director now, and the perpetrator is now only a character in your play.

GRATITUDE IN THE FORGIVENESS PROCESS

Gratitude is another novel component of forgiving, but you may be surprised to learn how I define gratitude. There are mental health professionals who teach you to forgive by expressing gratitude for the painful lesson you learned from your perpetrator. I consider this approach naive and damaging because, in addition to being irrelevant to forgiving, it implicitly views the perpetrator as a teacher. It's like thanking someone who rapes you for making you stronger and more sensitive to violence in the world. Not only does this approach increase your sense of victimhood, it also misunderstands the dynamics of healthy forgiveness. The gratitude I suggest you nurture has nothing to do with the predator and everything to do with rescuing your worthiness. I believe it is a revolutionary concept that requires careful scrutiny.

The best way for me to explain it is through another example. This time let's use forgiving a wound of abandonment. Your father left your family when you were twelve years old. You received no explanation and could find no apparent reason. You figured you had done something wrong, but you didn't know what it might have been, and your mother simply told you, "He wanted out."

This created a void, and you filled it with rationalizations and sadness. Since your mother remained in your life, it was easy to blame her.

(Children tend to blame the committed parent and excuse the irresponsible one.) Your feelings of unworthiness surfaced in the forms of poor academic performance, depression, and increased anger toward your mother. Since abandonment is the intimate language of love you learned when your father disappeared, you begin to abandon worthy goals, relationships, and ultimately your sense of purpose.

Years later, you reassess the circumstances of the abandonment and realize that your mother taught you commitment and your father abandonment. We learn good and bad lessons from deeds more than from words.

You also realize that you resent your dad for abandoning you, and feel guilty for your unjust anger toward your mother. You're ready to forgive, but when you try, your guilt over resenting your father and blaming your mother complicates the experiential process, and you end up settling for what I call *intellectual forgiveness:* a helpless imposition of mind over emotion. It doesn't work, and the unresolved wound continues to surface as self-sabotage whenever life offers you opportunities to prosper.

How can gratitude help? Could you be grateful to your mother for teaching you commitment by staying, or to your father for teaching you to overcome abandonment by leaving? Since biocognitive forgiveness has little to do with the perpetrator, let's find out why and how to correctly integrate gratitude into the experience of forgiveness.

I've explained throughout the book that emotions originating from love can recontextualize those coming from fear. We can change the felt meaning of fear in a context of love. Gratitude is an expression of love, and resentment a manifestation of fear, but I am not suggesting that shuffling these two emotions can resolve a grudge. In the example of abandonment, it would take more than replacing resentment with gratitude to recontextualize the felt meaning of the grudge.

Where you assign your gratitude rather than *how* you express it is what determines healthy resolution. The gratitude goes to *you* for continuing to live your honor, commitment, and loyalty despite your wound of shame, abandonment, or betrayal. One of the most important lessons here is that forgiveness is a liberation from the personal enslavement *you* construct when a misdeed is perpetrated against you. Rather than forgiving the perpetrator or minimizing the intensity of the misdeed, you recover the empowerment and self-worthiness you thought had been taken from you.

In other words, when you are wounded, you inadvertently offer ownership of your empowerment and worthiness to the perpetrator—even though the perpetrator is unaware of your offer because it takes place in your biocognitive space rather than outside of yourself. Thus, the liberation of forgiveness permits you to own empowerment and worthiness without involving the perpetrator at all; since the offer was never consummated, the perpetrator does not need to be involved in the recovery. In fact, even if the perpetrator accepted your offer, it would still be coauthored in your biocognitive space!

THE COMPONENTS OF A GRUDGE

I intentionally included *guilt* in the abandonment example to illustrate its relationship to *resentment* and how these two counterproductive emotions constitute a *grudge* when the misdeed was perpetrated by a cultural editor you love. A grudge becomes a circular loop of resentment and guilt; you feel resentment for the misdeed committed against you and guilt for resenting the perpetrator.

But how would this concept of a grudge work when it concerns the misdeeds of strangers? Would you feel guilty for resenting a stranger who maligned you? Perhaps not, but as time passes, you may notice that your resentment has turned into hatred, and that its intensity is limiting your ability to express love to your family. In this situation, you may feel guilty anyway—for neglecting people you love. Fortunately, the resentment and guilt that block forgiveness are resolved when you achieve liberation through an act of self-love.

The most significant lesson in this chapter is that you were never robbed of your power or your worthiness; you inadvertently disowned them. Similarly, honor, commitment, and loyalty were not lost when you were wounded; instead they remained hidden because you have not recognized your worthy deeds. Your capacity for self-love can be suppressed, but never stolen.

The Alpha Event

The mindbody forgiveness process has two sequential stages: the first reinstates your empowerment and the second your worthiness. When you recall and embody the felt meaning of the healing field that corresponds to your wound, you experience the *alpha event:* recognition of your goodness. This enables you to recover the sense of empowerment that has been depleted by the misdeed. Here's how the alpha event works:

* an archetypal wound challenges your vulnerability,
* unresolved vulnerability creates a sense of helplessness, and
* accessing the healing fields reinstates empowerment.

When you regain empowerment, you can release your victimhood. The healing fields involved (honor, commitment, and loyalty) do not need to be related to the misdeed or its perpetrator. The objective is to *recognize* that your empowerment was never lost; the misdeed compelled you to hide it, and evidence of your worthiness brings it back. Think of it this way: If someone tells you that you are unattractive, you can believe it until you look at yourself in the mirror and witness your beauty. It was never lost. It just remained dormant until you recognized it again. After you have recognized it, do you need permission from the other person to confirm what you observe? Of course not. This evidence-based recognition method illustrates that *you do not need to involve the perpetrator at all to confirm your worthiness.*

The Omega Event

In the alpha event you recognize your deeds of honor, commitment, and loyalty. In the *omega event,* you feel grateful for recognizing them. Recognition of your goodness reinstates your empowerment, and gratitude recovers your worthiness. Thus, as the director of your adapted play, you have changed the script that blocks your self-love. The alpha event begins your liberation, and the omega event completes it.

Disengaging the Perpetrator

Before you actually experience the forgiveness process yourself, it may seem that it will be incomplete because it works without engaging the perpetrator, so let me offer another analogy to further clarify. If some-one shot you in the shin, proper medical intervention would heal your gunshot wound. Would you have to forgive the person who shot you? No, you're not concerned with the shooter when you enter the emergency room. After treatment, your gunshot wound will heal independently of the person who shot you. You regain your power when you recognize the wound heals because of *your* immune system, and you feel worthy of heal-ing when you experience gratitude for seeking medical help, following postsurgery instructions, and having the internal resources to repair tissue.

Although I am using a physical instead of an emotional wound to explain a biocognitive process, the dynamics of how we relinquish our power and our worthiness—as well as how we sabotage our healing—are surprisingly similar in both circumstances. Rather than mind-body splitting, I propose mindbody integration. I can assure you that this forgiveness process works if you can suspend what you were taught about how to forgive. The old play of sympathy for the perpetrator is adapted when you write a new script offering empathy for yourself, the one who experienced the injury.

THE BIOCOGNITIVE PROCESS OF FORGIVENESS

Now it's time to learn how to experience forgiveness as liberation from self-entrapment. Depending on your cultural history, the intensity of your wound, and *your* conception of the perpetrator, the amount of time and effort needed to achieve forgiveness may vary. Be kind to your-self as you are learning these steps. If you are in therapy, continue your treatment as prescribed and let your health care professional help you enhance what you learn here. Most important, experience the process as the director of your newly adapted play.

<><><><><><><><><><><><><><><><><><><><><><><>

Confronting Your Grudge

❖ Following the usual method of becoming quiet
to start any biocognitive process, find a place

where you can sit and relax. Be aware of your
breathing and observe your inner world to quiet
your mind. If you notice any tension, observe
where and how it feels, without trying to
intervene in its unfolding.

❖ Identify what or whom you want to forgive,
replay the wounding incident as accurately
as possible, and observe your mindbody
manifestations. It helps if you can recall your
approximate age and the circumstance when the
incident took place.

❖ Identify the perpetrator and the wound you
experienced. Observe how your memories are
expressed in your mindbody. What thoughts,
sensations, and emotions do you feel?
Observe them as if you were watching clouds
passing by. Nonjudgmental observations
begin the healing process.

❖ Let the grudge surface and observe the anger,
resentment, and/or guilt it may bring to
awareness. The cluster of emotions may include
positive and mixed emotions. For example, love,
fear/love, resentment/love, resentment/guilt, and
so on. Do not try to interpret the emotions. Feel
them as they surface.

❖ Determine how you have used your grudge
to block your own liberation and used your
wound to gain sympathy. Observe how your
mindbody responds. Do not set expectations.
Your mindbody knows how to process emotions
without intellectual instructions.

Confronting Your Victimhood

❖ Imagine how you would live differently if you were to heal your wound. What would you have to give up, and how would you behave differently with others from a place of empowerment? Would you have to give up being excused for being moody or for not shouldering your fair share of responsibilities? Would you come out of your shell and become more involved with friends and family? Empowerment means having access to resources so you can meet challenges from strength, rather than having power over others through victimhood. Do not blame yourself; simply observe.

❖ Identify coauthors of your victimhood. Even if you do not feel you are using victimhood to gain power, allow yourself to explore the possibility.

❖ Recall situations when you allowed your coauthors to give you sympathy. How does it feel, and where does it manifest in your mindbody? Observe without judging yourself or your coauthors. If you can't recall any instance, continue to observe how you feel. Do you feel blocked? If you do, how does it manifest?

❖ Imagine what you can accomplish when you are empowered again, and what you can as a victim. If this does not apply to you, be creative and imagine a situation in which you could use victimhood to get what you want. Observe how the situation feels, and determine if it rings true.

The Alpha Event

❖ Recall memories of expressing your corresponding healing field: your honorable behavior if your wound is shame; your commitment if it's abandonment; your loyalty if it's betrayal. This is important: the incidents you call to mind do not need to be related to the misdeed in any way.

❖ Observe and experience your memories of healing fields. Although at the time they occurred, you did not interpret these empowering behaviors as such, you were intuitively attempting to compensate for your wound. What heals is the mindful recognition that you are the owner of these empowering deeds.

❖ Look for other healing-field deeds from your past. Again, they do not have to be associated with the wound and its circumstances. They are empowering independent of their association with the perpetrator. In addition to the healing field for your wound, you can also recall instances when you lived the other two healing fields.

❖ Observe and experience how other healing-field deeds manifest in your mindbody. Experiencing memories of any of the three healing fields can contribute to recognition of your worthiness.

❖ Allow yourself to experience the felt meaning and your ownership of these empowering deeds. For example, observe how it feels when you recognize that your empowerment was never lost. It was merely hidden from you by your wound.

❖ Identify coauthors in the present who would encourage your new, empowering awareness. Experience what you feel when you imagine sharing your new discoveries with them.

❖ Identify coauthors who would discourage your new, empowering awareness. Experience what you feel when you imagine sharing your new discoveries with them.

❖ Commit to continuing to recall incidents of healing-field deeds, and enact them in new situations in your life as much as you are able. Anytime you see the potential to fall into victimhood, explore ways to respond with healing-field behaviors. Honor, commitment, and loyalty become your new empowerment mindfulness.

◇◇◇◇◇◇◇◇◇◇◇◇◇◇◇◇◇◇◇◇◇◇◇

The Omega Event

❖ Recall your empowerment deeds again and experience their manifestations in your mindbody. Do they manifest in the same areas as before? Is their intensity different? Do you feel them differently?

❖ Extend gratitude to yourself for rescuing your empowerment. Be aware that sometimes gratitude surfaces as pride in your accomplishments. If this happens, let the experience unfold into gratitude. For example, if you feel proud of yourself for having been honorable, committed, or loyal, be thankful, and you'll notice how gratitude surfaces.

❖ When you feel gratitude, smile and allow all that
   is good about you to surface. The smile sends the
   message to your brain that you are open to recalling
   worthy memories.

❖ Repeat in your mind the words "thank you" like a
   mantra and embody their felt meaning. The thanking
   mantra is a way to reinforce gratitude or to facilitate
   recalling it. As you repeat the mantra, observe your
   mindbody without expectations. Remember, this
   process suspends judgment and lets your experiences
   unfold with healing strength.

❖ If you have difficulty experiencing gratitude or recalling
   healing-field deeds, observe how your mindbody
   experiences the difficulty. Repeat this question, "What
   is good about me?" Observe your mindbody rather
   than expect answers.

❖ Repeat the thanking mantra again and allow your
   mindbody to assimilate it. You will notice that any
   tightness you experience begins to melt, and you will
   be more accepting of your intention to feel grateful.

❖ Identify coauthors in the present who would celebrate
   your new gratitude mindfulness with you. Observe how
   it feels to imagine the celebration.

❖ If the perpetrator of the wound or the wound itself
   ever comes to awareness, observe the mindbody
   manifestations. Then celebrate your awareness of your
   empowering healing-field deeds and your gratitude for
   owning them. The wounds will heal and the perpetrator
   will be neutralized as you continue to confront fear
   with love.

❖ Permit your worthiness to surface from gratitude, and experience its newly felt meaning. For example, if you previously dismissed or rationalized your good deeds, now you can allow them to surface without interpreting their meaning and with gratitude for your observations (good or bad).

❖ Commit to experiencing gratitude for any healing-field deeds you do, and find other creative ways to acknowledge you worthiness. Anytime there is a potential to fall into unworthiness, explore ways to respond with gratitude for any recent accomplishments. Let honor, commitment, and loyalty become your new worthiness mindfulness.

<><><><><><><><><><><><><>

Reconciliation

❖ Determine whether you want to reconcile with your perpetrator. Observe your mindbody reaction. Would you do it to be accepted? To be liked? Because they are family? Remember, reconciliation is not necessary unless you decide it's in the best interest of your wellness. It should never be based on victimhood or done at your own expense.

❖ If you decide not to reconcile, be grateful to yourself for making this decision. Do not expect your perpetrator to like it. If you experience sympathy for your perpetrator, remember that you are really offering pity. Pity is not a healthy emotion for you or the other person. Instead, allow your decision to be experienced with self-love.

❖ If you decide to reconcile, set limits. The reconciliation should be empowering for you. You can set limits for the conditions of your contact with this person, such as frequency, duration, and whether others are present. Liberating yourself from self-entrapment does not mean the perpetrator has become a better person.

❖ If you decide to reconcile with a family member who is toxic, determine how much time and frequency they can handle before their toxicity surfaces. For example, if you decide to reconcile with a toxic mother, give her the dosage of love *she* can tolerate without becoming toxic or wounding you again.

◇◇◇◇◇◇◇◇◇◇◇◇◇◇

Redemption

❖ Redemption should only be exercised if what you are redeeming enhances your worthiness. For example, if after recontextualizing your wound and experiencing your liberation, you realize you were unfair in your assessment of the wounding, own up to your misinterpretation and determine whether the perpetrator is worthy of redemption. The best apology is empathic action.

❖ If *you* decide redemption is not an empowering and worthy option, let the person go. If they are family you still love, love them from a distance and celebrate having known what was good about them.

❖ ❖ ❖

I hope you can see now why I shared so much information before teaching you this deep and powerful experiential process. Like all biocognitive methods, the forgiveness process you learned is indirect and counter-intuitive, but powerful in the way it liberates you from self-entrapment without involving the perpetrator of your wounds. By the way, if you are wondering how to forgive yourself for perpetrating your own wounds, I have good news for you; you can use the same forgiveness process because the dynamics do not change. Whether you wound yourself or allow others to wound you, forgiving is an act of self-love that will allow you to regain the empowerment and worthiness that has merely been hidden from view, never lost.

9

Psychospiritual Conflicts
and Their Resolutions

I
n this chapter, I will introduce you to an emerging field of applied theology
called *contemplative psychology,* a new discipline that brings together the
best of Western and Eastern mystical-theology models of inquiry to explore
how spiritual beliefs affect physical and mental health. More important, this
chapter deals with what I call *psychospiritual conflicts,* how they can mimic
psychiatric disorders, and how to address the root of this problem.

The unique contribution of contemplative psychology to our understanding of theology as a belief system is that, rather than studying
religions with a particular psychological orientation, it studies the
psychology within each religion. For example, instead of examining
Buddhism from psychoanalytical or other theoretical perspectives, it
studies the psychology embedded in the teachings of Buddhism itself.
This method allows us to extract the psychological value of a theological
model without any preconceived notions.

From the beginning, I want to be clear that my objective in this
chapter is to show that we experience metaphysical beliefs—whether
about God, nature, or any other entity—with our mindbody, and consequently, this affects our biology. In fact, even atheists are affected by their
belief because believing that something does not exist is still a belief. So
whether you are religious, spiritual, or atheist, I invite you to enter this
area of inquiry with an open mind.

THE POWER OF OUR BELIEFS

What we choose to believe affects how we deal with our world, and we construct our "world" based on what we perceive with our culturally trained brain. So what is reality? It depends on your perceptual equipment and your cultural history.

When you look at a sunflower, you see shades of yellow and orange within the range between infrared and ultraviolet that your human vision permits. But if a bee looks at the same sunflower, it sees ultraviolet colors, and a snake sees infrared. Did the sunflower change? Obviously not; it simply coauthored the perceiver's "reality" based on perceptual capabilities. Although I am not a reductionist, as a scientist I do admit that we are limited by our physical makeup. *But* our thoughts, dreams, and beliefs transcend that physical makeup. And although we do our thinking within our biological body, we are more than a body. The moment we engage a belief, it transforms into something *other* than the body in which it was coauthored.

Paradoxically, although a belief is not "physical," it can affect our physical body. When the entities we call beliefs relate to the existence of something beyond our physicality, they enter a dimension I call *psychospiritual*, which includes spiritual, religious, and theological beliefs as well as any other conception of existence beyond our physical life.

How Your Beliefs Affect Your Health and Longevity

Believing you are loved, whether or not you are actually loved, positively affects your health and longevity. Conversely, believing you are not loved—true or not—negatively affects your health and longevity. I have witnessed the first in my investigations of centenarians, and the second in patients who cannot heal, independent of medical intervention, because of their lack of self-love. You can also see how lack of self-love affects longevity in the high incidence of death by suicide and overdose among superstars. Although they are loved and admired by millions, their lack of self-love does not permit them to reap the benefits of that love.

But how can a nonphysical entity affect our health and longevity? Rather than going into heavy philosophical inquiry, let's bring biocognitive science to the rescue.

Mind and body are inseparable. Our biology creates thoughts, and our thoughts create biology; we coauthor our *mindbodyness*. The belief that we can separate our mind from our body is, like any other belief, an inseparable mindbody process. Thus, rather than trying to separate mind from body, let's explore beliefs as mindbody expressions that, because they are inseparable, affect each other.

Of course, you know by now that you sometimes may get a little dizzy as I prepare you for the main course, but I hope that by this stage of your journey through the book, you can see it more as a necessary stage of preparation than as an annoyance. I respect your intelligence and appreciate the opportunity you are giving me to share my work with you, so I want to dig deeply into the concepts I am proposing, anticipate your questions and doubts, and leave you with a substantive understanding.

Just as believing you are loved is good for you, independent of confirmation that you are loved, studies show that having spiritual beliefs positively affects your health. Here, I am reminded of Pascal's wager: whether God exists or not, there is more benefit and less harm in believing in him than in not.

Although Pascal's wager was quite clever, let me clarify the condition he proposed. Studies show that people who believe in God and attend regular religious services with family have better health and longevity than nonbelievers. But let's go deeper. Other studies demonstrate that the benefits only extend to those who believe in a god of love, rather than a wrathful god. There are other, nonspiritual factors here that we need to include in our inquiry. You can experience psychoneuroimmunological benefits by believing in a loving entity, whether that entity exists or not. And any loving ritual, religious or not, performed with family has wellness benefits. Social psychology research adds one more factor: people who regularly worship with family are less likely to engage in risky or harmful behavior. Does this mean one causes the other? No; they share coauthorship.

THE FOUR STAGES OF CHANGE

Since the beginning of my career in clinical neuropsychology, I've been fascinated by the complexity involved in individual change. What makes people implement changes that improve their quality of life? More important, what stops them from changing what does not serve them well? In some extreme cases, even being fully aware that not changing can kill you is not sufficient to inspire the change. Sadly, I have seen patients who choose to die when their cure requires angering others. After years of frustrated attempts to help others change what ails them, I finally found the four sequential stages of change.

Most minor conditions can be resolved in the first and second stages, most mindbody change requires the first three stages, and psychospiritual change can only happen when the cycle is complete at the fourth stage. For this chapter, I will concentrate on this fourth stage, not only because it has to do with spirituality, but because unresolved spiritual conflict can mimic psychiatric illness. In other words, some illnesses can be mindbody expressions of spiritual conflict.

To create a visual example using the configuration of each term, imagine the hyphenated word *mind-body-spirit* representing the split that causes illness, and *mindbodyspirit* illustrating the fusion of the three when healing takes place.

Stage One: Behavior Change

Most change can take place at this stage without having to involve the other three: for example, changing the way you comb your hair, your food preferences, your exercise routine, and so on. But I will use alcohol addiction as an example to illustrate what takes place at each of the four stages.

When the alcoholic stops drinking, the change occurs at the behavioral level (from drinking to not drinking). But we know that behavioral change, while necessary, is not sufficient to resolve addictions. Yet unfortunately, some people stop at this stage and assume their change is complete.

Stage Two: Meaning Change

Here you identify the meaning that drives the behavior and its function. The alcoholic has to determine what the drinking behavior allows and what it avoids. Excessive drinking may facilitate facing an angry partner without feeling much pain and avoiding *meaningful* conversation during dinner.

Nothing changes after the drinking stops (stage one) unless there is recognition that the drinking has a function other than getting drunk (stage two). If this second stage of change is not completed, the drinking will continue or will be replaced with another form of avoidance, such as overworking, gambling, or anything else that continues to accomplish what drinking does.

Stage Three: Confronting Coauthors and Environments

Let's assume the alcoholic stops drinking and recognizes the functional meaning of the alcoholic behavior. Then comes confronting what or who has been coauthoring the avoidance. Most patients who discontinue therapy do so at this stage to avoid the inevitable confrontation with their coauthors. Stage three requires changing responses to old patterns; for the alcoholic, this may entail confronting fear and a partner without being inebriated. Stage three is also difficult for the coauthors because their old ways of responding to the alcoholic also need to change. Sometimes coauthors sabotage the change to avoid their own dysfunctional issues. Addictions *always* involve codependence.

So far, these first three stages are not monumental news. Most people implicitly understand the reasons why these steps are necessary for change. Stage four, however, is the most difficult because it involves psychospiritual conflict.

Stage Four: Spiritual Resolution

The first three stages of change are shaped by cultural beliefs; they involve what your culture determines is acceptable behavior, the punishment for noncompliance, and how to correct unwanted behavior. Stage four is different. It has to do with the spiritual or religious beliefs you developed regarding your transcendental options, your transgressions, and your deity. What if an alcoholic is able to work through the first three stages but comes from a psychospiritual belief system that teaches that alcohol consumption is a mortal sin *without redemption?*

This psychospiritual impasse is not limited to addicts. I had a patient who went through frequent psychotic episodes despite taking antipsychotic medication. We could not figure out what was happening until I asked him about his religious beliefs. He told me he had given up on his religion and was not interested in discussing it. Here is an illustration of the importance of digging deeper: I found out from his wife—his third wife—that he came from a fundamentalist religion that considers divorce a mortal sin punishable by eternal damnation. In other words, although he thought he had dismissed his psychospiritual upbringing, his psychosis made it clear that his mindbodyspirit did not agree.

I persuaded the patient to consider that his psychospiritual conflict was mimicking a psychiatric illness. What could we do? We brought to our interdisciplinary treatment team a theologian from the patient's religious denomination, someone who was well respected (a cultural editor) and who could offer an empathic interpretation of its sacred scriptures.

Prior to our intervention, the patient's first divorce had been the beginning of his psychospiritual damnation. His psychosis ruined his second marriage and was about to destroy his third, when we treated him with a different model. The result? After additional interdisciplinary therapy, he was taken off medications and continues to do well with his third wife. Such cases of psychospiritual conflict mimicking psychiatric illness are not frequently found in medical literature, not because they are rare but because they are misdiagnosed as psychiatric disorders—the psychospiritual dimension is not addressed.

THE TRANSCENDENTAL DECISION

The ultimate reality is that we are aware of our mortality. I strongly argue that whether we believe we transcend our physical existence in a spiritual afterlife, reincarnate, or simply end as biodegradable material, we need to resolve our existential despair. We all experience it when we think of our end or witness someone else's. Just as we find meaning in our daily existence, we can bring meaning to our end.

Independent of what you think happens after your physical life ends, all your assumptions are based on faith: a choice to believe or disbelieve, without evidence. Since you can construct whatever personal cosmology you choose, why not choose one that brings you serenity? But after you do comes the most important question: how do you live your life after choosing a cosmology of your end?

Some religious leaders are convinced that religion can help contain the savage within through fear of eternal damnation. Others propose that life has no meaning without a belief in the existence of God. In my view, these unresolved issues beg these questions: Are we good because we fear eternal punishment? Do we love because we fear existential loneliness? Can we endure life if we know there is nothing beyond it?

Contemplative psychology offers effective methods to navigate and resolve our existential despair. More important, serenity is available independent of the cosmology we choose to endorse. Before moving on with our psychospiritual exploration, I will share my personal beliefs—without any intention to influence yours.

I *choose* to believe that we are much more than biochemical accidents and evolutionary machines. But this belief is not based on fear of an afterlife reprisal at the hands of a punitive deity. If God exists, it must be pure love. I'd rather burn in hell than worship a wrathful entity. But there is no need to get melodramatic here—I am leading up to the most important component of building your personal cosmology if you don't have one.

Independent of your belief in an afterlife, you must decide if you are going to base your existence on love or fear. I have known compassionate atheists and malicious believers. I have treated murderers, rapists, and serial killers whose behavior was never stopped by fear of spiritual damnation. In fact, some continued their inhumane behavior because they believed that since they had been irreversibly damned after they committed their first act of infamy, they had free rein now, with no additional punitive consequences.

Something else I discovered while doing contemplative psychology workshops is also worth mentioning. During the experiential exercises involved, some people realized they had accepted neatly packaged transcendental beliefs from their spiritual authorities without the opportunity to contribute to their own cosmology. Toward the end of the chapter, I'll teach you a method to assess your transcendental beliefs and explore possible modifications of them based on your personal preferences. If you are comfortable with your transcendence model, you can skip that part, or you can learn it so you can teach it to others who may need it.

MYSTICAL SCIENTIST VERSUS SCIENTIFIC MYSTIC

The notion of the mystical scientist versus the scientific mystic is not mine, but I can't recall the originator to give him or her credit. What I'll share here is my interpretation of those two options as additional tools for your journey. But you need be neither a mystic nor a scientist to benefit from this inquiry. Science gives facts, and spirituality gives profound meaning. Scientists rely on measurements, and mystics are guided by their inner voice. Christian mystics seek unity with God; Buddhist mystics seek oneness with all. Western mystics live to learn through suffering, and Eastern mystics live to end suffering. Although I am generalizing, when you look into the lives of mystics across cultures, you can differentiate their concepts of suffering by their Eastern or Western cosmologies.

Adapting the multitasking style of modern life, I offer two effective paths of inquiry to cut through external distractions and find mindbodyspirit serenity. When I speak of mysticism, I am not referring to the magical and esoteric concepts promoted by New Age teachers. Instead, I refer to professional theologians trained in using the contemplative methods of their respective religions to find God or oneness with whatever may be considered divine. One of my mentors, Father Jack Finnegan, a pioneer of contemplative psychology, defines mysticism as "applied theology." Father Finnegan is an Irish psychologist and Catholic priest who taught me some of the contemplative psychology lessons I am sharing with you.

If you choose the mystical scientist approach, your life is guided by your inner voice to find meaning in your external world. If you choose the way of the scientific mystic, you are guided by your external world to find meaning in your inner voice. Let's unravel these concepts with examples.

In my view, Einstein was a scientific mystic. His discoveries of relativity and how gravity is created by the bending of space gave him internal meaning. Conversely, Nelson Mandela was a mystical scientist. He was guided by his inner voice of compassion to create the Truth and Reconciliation Commission that prevented genocide in South Africa after the end of apartheid. Although neither of these figures was a mystic, they each found meaning from different perspectives. In the practical applications section at the end of this chapter, I'll teach you how to navigate your chosen path to find your internal meaning.

CONTEMPLATIVE METHODS OF INQUIRY

I cannot overemphasize the importance of understanding that contemplative psychology is a science of mind-in-the-world. It is not a religion or a selection of one theology over another. Rather than being an intellectual exercise, contemplative methods inquire with the mind embodied in experience.

Mystics from all five major world religions use some form of contemplation to reach the deepest level of union with their god or divine essence. Whether you are Christian, Muslim, Jewish, Hindu, Buddhist, or atheist, you can use contemplative methods to understand the essence of compassion or any other human attribute. But before you can enter deeper levels of contemplation, you need three tools to free yourself from ego attachments, cultural biases, political correctness, and other *discursive noise* (jumping from thought to thought, subject to subject, and so on).

Father Finnegan calls these three methods of inquiry *Greek cognitive tools* because Aristotle and others before him used them to identify and navigate the *contemplative labyrinth*. Consider the significance of what we are about to do: apply the tools of the greatest philosophers of ancient Greece to help us decipher the same challenges they encountered more than 2,200 years ago.

Apophasis

Apophasis is the first contemplative tool. The Greek word literally means "to say no." You are saying no to the language and imagery that block your transcendence into undisturbed experience. For example, if you apply the apophatic method to knowing the wind, you begin by negating the attributes you give the wind: wind is not a thing, wind is not movement, wind is not space, and so on, until you reach a point where you exhaust all your intellectual associations with the subject of inquiry. You are left with a space void of words and imagery.

The apophatic method applied to knowing God would be this: God is not omnipotent, not compassionate, not omnipresent, and so on. But it's important to understand that this negation is not to deny existence or to be negative. It is a way of intuiting that God is more than we can embrace with words. God is beyond description.

The apophatic method is also used in Zen Buddhist koans, riddles that cannot be solved using language or logic. Koans can be riddles, such as "What is the color of the wind?" or "What is Zen?" Their purpose is to test the depth of your understanding and help you realize that language and logic will not work. Instead, you eventually reach insight into the nature of the question without necessarily being able to describe it directly with words. In addition to the apophatic method, Zen koans also use paradox to create what is called the Great Doubt; for example, "What is the compassion of hatred?" This method of inquiry also helps you recognize that there are other dimensions of experience beyond descriptive language.

Aphaeresis

After you say no to language and imagery, *aphaeresis* (literally "to let go") is the tool that releases them. Apophasis refuses the blocks—distractions to avoid going deeper—and aphaeresis gets rid of them. In your contemplative inquiry, you can negate the cultural and egoist associations blocking what you are trying to know at its essence, but then you have to learn ways to let go of the blocks. Staying in the apophatic stage will only rerun your "not" statements without extracting them from your contemplative path.

For example, you recognize that you're not a bad person, but you continue to helplessly function as if you were. In this case, you are saying no without releasing the culprit—out of sight, out of mind. These contemplative tools clarify why changing what does not serve us well requires more than recognizing the damage. In fact, I have used these contemplative tools to help addicts identify and release the sociocultural distractions that maintain their addictions. But the next tool is the most difficult to implement because it requires navigating the experiential vacuum that is created when you remove the blocks.

Aporia

Aporia is the tool that helps you reach what is not possible with linguistic inquiry. The Greek word means "without way or passage." The explanation gets a bit tricky because I must necessarily describe with words an experience that transcends language. Here again, I will rely on what I learned from Father Finnegan to explain it. Perhaps I can do this by talking around it using his method of poetics—imaginative and speculative reflection to illustrate a contemplation that does not have imagery and does not speculate.

How's that for paradox? Once more, I trust your curiosity and intellect to enter where others fear to tread.

Aporia suspends cognition with a startling flash of perplexity and opens a portal to navigate a spiritual dimension from the perspective of contemplative theology—or noncontextual consciousness, from the approach of neuroscience. Whether the objective is to find God or explore the deepest layer of consciousness, the three Greek tools can teach you the way. What is most interesting to me is that both spiritual and secular seekers describe this state of *suspended knowing* in remarkably similar ways: profound peace, boundless love, oneness, infinite compassion, and other poignant qualities that can only be approximated with language. Not bad results, whether you're spiritual or not!

More important for our objectives in this chapter, this exalted experience triggers powerful psychopharmacological effects that can only enhance the treatment of psychiatric disorders. Just as psychospiritual conflict can mimic psychiatric disturbances, deep contemplative states of what Buddhists call *lovingkindness* can actually shift activity from the brain's right prefrontal lobe to the left, increasing serotonin, dopamine, and other neurotransmitters as effectively as psychotropic medication. But let me be clear: I am *not* suggesting replacing medication with contemplation to treat psychiatric disorders. Instead, I believe nonpharmacological tools that affect brain chemistry in the desired direction can be incorporated with conventional psychiatric protocols. I predict, however, that as we learn more about how to affect brain chemistry with mindbody methods, some pharmaceutical companies will have to look for other ways to generate revenue.

THE THREE GREEK TOOLS APPLIED TO MINDFULNESS

I am going to assume you are coming from one of two perspectives: either a spiritual one, or one of wanting to learn more about contemplative neuroscience without concern for spirituality. The tools work equally well for both. What I don't want to do is make either condition a requirement for benefiting from the information I am sharing in this chapter. Both pursuits are most welcome.

In chapter 10, I will explain mindfulness and mindlessness from the perspectives of contemplative science and social psychology. Here I'll use the three Greek tools to inquire into mindfulness itself. In other words, instead of looking at mindfulness as a tool, let's use these three contemplative tools to inquire into the essence of mindfulness. Think of it as putting on a pair of glasses so you can find your other pair.

The Apophatic Tool—Mindfulness is not thoughts, not logic, not interpretation, not description, not purpose, not expectation, not emotions, and so on. Here you exhaust your associations and categories, but they keep spinning when you try to move on.

The Aphaeresis Tool—So, if mindfulness is not any of the things you think it is, what the hell is it? The what-the-hell-is-it question *is* the blocking agent to be released with this tool. Blocks are premises that generate all the incessant categorizing that goes on in your head. In other words, all the attempts to define and encapsulate your thinking are based on one premise: you must label things in order to understand them. The aphaeresis tool gets rid of that premise, and the labeling stops.

The Aporia Tool—When you remove noise from the inquiry, it creates a cognitive vacuum. It can be very perplexing because you are introduced to *meaningless wisdom*. But terms are misunderstood when you use descriptive language to explain contemplative experiences. In other words, in semantics, the term *meaningless* is another way of describing nonsense, irrelevance, and lack of value.

So how can wisdom be meaningless? Because words can only be defined by other words, so you can't explain deeper levels of consciousness without creating contradictions. To further complicate the inquiry, when you also remove images, you end up with what contemplatives call *meaningful nothingness.* The point here is that the vacuum you navigate with aporia can only be described linguistically with poetics, paradox, or oxymoron. Perplexed? If you are, congratulations—you've just encountered the Great Doubt. The tools that serve you well to communicate and understand the "world out there" no longer work when you navigate the vastness of your inner wisdom. The good news is that there is no deeper meaning and no greater serenity than the dimension where aporia takes you.

CONTEMPLATIVE KNOWING

When we want to know something, we assume one language of inquiry fits all. We apply this language to communicate and gather knowledge in the "world out there." Since it works well, we learn to trust it and continue to use it. We also learn to trust strategies that worked well in the past, and we use them with the expectation that they will not disappoint us. Then, when we encounter transcendental questions and profound existential challenges, we apply our trusted language and strategies—but to our dismay, they don't work. Why not? What are we doing wrong? Let's look for answers.

There are three languages of inquiry, each with a range of functions: *descriptive, prescriptive,* and *evocative.* Their names illustrate what they do. To cover a wide range of subjects, let's use a mundane and a profound example: knowing an apple and knowing God.

The descriptive language teaches you apples are red and round; prescriptive explains you can eat them raw or cooked; but evocative must be experienced because it awakens (evokes) a particular state of reality in which description and prescription will not suffice. When you hold and taste an apple, it *evokes* flavor, aroma, roundness, heft, and so on. In biocognition terms, the evocative language illustrates the experience of coauthoring within a bioinformational field. Some contemplatives call it communing with the evoked.

Now, moving from the profane to the divine: descriptively, God is omnipotent; prescriptively, God is to be loved; evocatively, God is . . . ? You don't *know* until you commune with what God evokes. Contemplative inquiry provides evocative language to know God. But not forgetting those who are seeking oneness rather than divinity, the same principles of contemplative inquiry can be applied to communing with nature or your own essence. This is what the often abused and misunderstood term *oneness* means when you rescue it from the platitudes of gurus, the usual suspects who offer *nothing* rather than *nothingness*. I also want to clarify that spirituality is not restricted to seeking God. For example, Buddhism is a profoundly spiritual *and* godless religion. Whether you seek God, Self, Nature, or atheism, the contemplative path can teach you how to commune with the essence of whatever you seek.

Han de Wit, a foremost scholar of contemplative psychology, suggests contemplative traditions are primarily interested in producing competent knowers rather than knowledge.

It reminds me of what my martial arts teacher asked me when I won my black belt in Tae Kwon Do: "What does the black belt mean to you?"

In my ego-based, prescriptive language, I answered, "It means I am highly skilled in the martial arts."

He corrected me with the kick of Great Doubt, "No. Now, you're a serious student."

As novices, we begin the contemplative inquiry with our egos because it is very enticing to apply familiar tools to solving unfamiliar challenges. But when we experience the limitations of our knowledge, the contemplative path provides an opportunity to become a better knower.

THE UNDULATIONS OF KNOWING

Saint Teresa of Avila was a sixteenth-century Catholic nun who is considered one the most prolific mystics and contemplative scholars of Christian theology. In her *prayer of quiet,* which is a contemplative method and not a prayer, she warns that God cannot be known with our faculties (cognition) because we are not prepared to handle the intensity of the experience. The prayer of quiet teaches you to drop your ego and create a *place of quiet* where God can bestow his wisdom. But the objective is to invite God to the place of quiet, not to seek him.

This contemplative path is beneficial whether you seek God or inner peace. In modern psychological language, the prayer of quiet teaches you to drop sociocultural assumptions and explore noncontextual mindbody states. When Tibetan lamas and other highly skilled meditators are in deep contemplation, they produce gamma brain waves, indicating a state of extraordinary mindbody cohesiveness—an ideal condition for mindfulness learning. Gamma brain waves are rare and not produced readily. They can be incidentally generated in Saint Teresa's metaphorical place of quiet. Of course, gamma rhythms come from the hippocampus, the part of the brain associated with memory during concentration and learning.

And now, to anticipate concerns about recent research showing that rats increase gamma activity in the hippocampus when they are forced to run quickly, do not worry about reductionist arguments against the value of contemplative methods. Since the hippocampus keeps track of where you are and when you change position, the rats' increased running speed required a faster rate of learning to remember quick changes in time and space. In other words, the rats needed increases in gamma activity to help them remember how to change positions rapidly. Rats learning how to run back and forth quickly in order to get food rewards is not the same as you knowing God—it is vastly different from contemplative states to know divinity or the essence of oneness. I should mention that the researchers in that study did not imply the rats' learning was any more than as I just described it.

If the contemplative methods use evocative language to teach you how to be a better knower rather than how to accumulate knowledge, then you can only *know* the evocations of the source. For example, rather than accumulating knowledge of God, you can only know the evocations you experience in unity with God. This is precisely what mystics from different theological perspectives conclude.

Let me use analogy to make this concept more understandable. When you throw a stone into a lake, the stone sinks, and all you see are ripples. You, the stone, and the lake have coauthored the ripples. Since evocative language connects you with the evocations (ripples) of the source, and not the source, I call it *undulations of knowing*—it awakens a state of reality beyond what descriptive and prescriptive language can achieve. For example, the undulations of knowing an apple are the taste, aroma, and heft it evokes, but since you can't use your senses to know the metaphysical, the undulations are intuited rather than perceived. You *know*, but words become awkward approximations when you describe what you learned.

THE CONTEMPLATIVE EXPERIENCE

Although the main objective of this chapter is to show you that contemplative psychology offers tools to resolve psychospiritual conflicts that mimic some psychiatric disorders, its methodologies can be applied with equal effectiveness to finding oneness with what you consider sacred or whose essence is worthy of knowing. Let's begin the experience.

<><><><><><><><><><><><><><><><><><><><><><>

Fourth Level Change

Since the first three levels of change are straightforward, and I have described their components in this and other chapters, I will now teach you the exercise for the fourth level of change.

If you completed the first two levels of change—the behavior, meaning, and function of a problem—and confronted and resolved any issues with your coauthors (level three), but you continue to have related symptoms (anxiety, depression, fear, and so on), you can go to the fourth level of change and see whether the conflict is psychospiritual. This exercise should not replace professional help, but it can enhance your treatment.

❖ Find time and a quiet place to relax and slow down your mind. Breathe and observe what is going on. Do not interpret what you find.

❖ Identify what model of retribution you were taught by the editors of your religion to deal with wrongdoing or sins. Were you taught to believe in God and afterlife judgment? Is it a loving or a wrathful god? Who taught you?

❖ Do you associate your symptoms with a sinful action or serious violation of your religious beliefs? If not, you can stop this exercise and move to the next section. If you identify a connection between your symptoms and fourth level change, continue.

❖ What punishment comes to mind when you identify your wrongful action? Do you consider it a mortal sin or something that clergy from your religion can help you resolve? Do you believe you should be punished? Are you punishing yourself?

❖ Identify what you feel and its mindbody manifestations. Observe and keep breathing slowly and deeply. See the manifestations as clouds that pass by.

❖ Find clergy from your religion who are willing to work with you to resolve your conflict at the psychospiritual level.

❖ Permit yourself to consider that there is a compassionate alternative to the punishment you were taught to associate with your wrongdoing. You can take responsibility for your wrongdoing and resolve it by making restitution rather than by making yourself sick.

❖ Bring to mind any act of compassion you have enacted for yourself or others. Recall something you did with kindness and empathy for yourself or others. Experience the mindbody reaction. Let it grow.

❖ Allow your mindbody to quiet by paying attention to what the compassionate memory evokes. From that mindbody state of self-compassion, decide what positive action you can take as restitution. For example, you can decide to do anonymous compassionate deeds. But do not do the action out of guilt or fear. Restitution includes reclaiming your worthiness.

❖ Once you commit to the restitution you have chosen, commune with your God or your divinity and offer it without expecting to understand the process or receive a response. You do this in the place of quiet you create to commune with the undulations of the source.

❖ After you complete the exercise, decide when you are going to implement your restitution. Do not wait long to implement it. You can also discuss it with your clergy.

❖ Look for undulations of love. For example, anytime you feel good about yourself, or someone does something kind for you, or you witness any act of kindness, view it as undulations conveying that your restitution is accepted by the source. The source could be God, nature, honor, compassion, and so on.

❖ Look for new opportunities where you can commune with gratitude. Whatever evokes gratitude within you, contextualize it as undulations of love from the source you sought to bring about fourth-order change. Be at peace with yourself. Your redeeming actions are not payment for your wrongdoing; they are expressions of lovingkindness transformed from guilt.

The Contemplative Method

❖ Use any of the quieting techniques from this book, or use your own, to slow your mindbody speed and noise. Breathe naturally and allow yourself to enter a place of serenity.

❖ After you reach a deep level of relaxation, subvocally say no to distracting thoughts and sensations. The apophasis method does not involve blocking. (The next step will clarify my point.)

❖ When a distraction enters, do not try to block it. Observe it and say, "Not me." For example, you are distracted with a thought about paying a bill. You say, "Not me," as you exhale with the distraction. You are beginning to detach from your thoughts. You are not your thoughts.

❖ Repeat this apophatic technique for a few minutes. Next, apply the aphaeresis tool of letting go.

❖ After subvocally saying, "Not me," pay attention to the period of nonthoughts that follows until another distraction surfaces. You are observing the silence that follows after you say, "Not me."

❖ When the nonthought period starts, say, "Not me" to the nonthought period as well. By detaching from the thought and the nonthought, you accomplish the aphaeresis technique of letting go. It is subtle and indirect.

❖ Continue to let go and observe how the nonthought segments get longer as the frequency and duration of distractions shorten. After you sense you are ready to move on, go to the next step: navigating the *without way* using aporia.

❖ Now, inhale with your awareness on *empty space* and exhale with it on *empty space.* In other words, imagine inhaling and exhaling from your nonthought space instead of from your chest and stomach.

❖ Continue this *analogous* breathing method for a few minutes. You will be able to do it very convincingly and sooner than you may expect. This relocated sensation begins the navigation of aporia: movement through nonthought space.

❖ Imagine that this nonthought process creates the place of quiet where deep truth is found, and divinity endows you with wisdom. In the quiet place you learn to be a better knower.

❖ Now remove your awareness from breathing, and stay in that quiet place, trusting your breathing to keep you there without awareness of the breath. This is a leap of faith. You are receptive to emptiness.

❖ Stay lost in that empty space of quiet for as long as you wish, and when you are ready to end the experience, return your awareness to your breathing, and slowly end the exercise.

❖ When you open your eyes, do not interpret what happened. You entered the quiet place with the evocative language to commune with evoked meaningless wisdom in meaningful nothingness. In other words, the quiet place evokes nothingness

to commune with it. Experience it without trying
to make sense of the process.

❖ Practice this contemplative method with regularity as a
new ritual, as well as when you need inner wisdom to
deal with external turbulence, psychospiritual conflict,
and any major challenge in life. Do not analyze the
experience. Communing with nothingness makes no
sense. That is how you create the quiet place.

The reason why it's counterproductive to analyze and try to
make sense of contemplative experiences is that you use linear
descriptive and prescriptive languages to understand nonlinear
evocative processes. It would be like concluding that the
ripple *is* the rock. As you practice these apparently simplistic
methods, you will become a better knower of your essence,
your cosmology, and the "world out there."

❖ ❖ ❖

In the next chapter, I'll teach you why wishful thinking followed by positive action is necessary but not sufficient to achieve sustainable change.
But for now, I will leave you with a quote from one of the foremost
masters of forgiveness, Nelson Mandela.

No one is born hating another person because of the color of
his skin, or his background, or his religion. People must learn
to hate, and if they can learn to hate, they can be taught to
love, for love comes more naturally to the human heart than
its opposite.

From Wishful Thinking
to Sustainable Action

THE ANTHROPOLOGY OF CAUSE AND EFFECT

Research in mindbody disciplines, such as psychoneuroimmunology and cultural neuroscience, is beginning to clarify why it is that wishful thinking, appealing to reason, and disembodied guided imagery have limited effects on changing our dysfunctional behavioral patterns. Biocognitive theory and practice offer a missing component: *you cannot sustain positive mindbody change unless you have a fundamental sense of self-worth that enables you to accept the benefits you can gain from the change.*

According to biocognitive theory, our perceptions are culturally learned. When we are confronted with challenging conditions—whether positive or negative—we respond with culturally learned interpretations that lead us to either feelings of empowerment or feelings of helplessness. And the cultural beliefs we apply to interpreting our challenges have horizons that expand or contract based on our level of self-worth. When we are confronted with turbulence in our lives, whether good or bad, we assume a cause and determine its effect based on our cultural history. In other words, the tribes in which we live teach us to assign certain causes to our circumstances and to respond in preset ways. A good example of this is that Americans from economically deprived families who win the lottery lose their fortune, on average, within eighteen months. They were taught that wealth is not an option.

In contrast, the biocognitive model of cause and effect is deceptively simple because what may seem mundane has deep implications for our cultural learning of self-valuation.

Since your culture originally taught you the causes you assign to your challenges and the strategies you choose to resolve the turbulence that accompanies them, you can also learn to recontextualize the felt meaning of turbulence as a potential opportunity to celebrate what you discover. Such mindbody changes require more than wishful thinking. You must recontextualize the felt meaning of the cultural symbols you ascribe to your challenges before you can consider alternative causes and solutions.

A concrete example will clarify the concept of cause and effect I am introducing here. Suppose you're promoted to a new position that comes with a substantial salary increase. Also suppose that your cultural editors have taught you to devalue your abilities and deny your accomplishments. The most likely reason or cause for your promotion that you will choose, then, is that you were "lucky." Since luck is an external factor you can't control, your response to your good fortune will probably be to worry about how long you will be on the job before your new boss notices your inadequacies. Your culture has taught you to feel unworthy, so not only do you credit luck rather than your own abilities for this new development, but you also choose to deal with it by investing your energy in expectations of catastrophe.

It is important to note that when you choose cause and effect in this way, you also assume others will come to the same conclusions. In this example, you assume your new boss can only conclude you lack the abilities to do the job. We project our beliefs in this way because we assume that others share them.

At the end of this chapter, I will show you how to recontextualize cause and effect.

COAUTHORING YOUR WORTHINESS

You can now recognize that your cultural editors taught you to interpret the causes and effects of events in your life, and you know why you project your interpretations onto others—you assume others see things as you do. When you realize that projection is a two-way street, you can begin to appreciate that coauthoring is a complex exchange of cultural perceptions. You project your interpretations of cause and effect onto your coauthors, and they reciprocate by projecting their own. I never cease to be amazed by how well we can communicate with our coauthors, despite our tendency to compare apples and oranges. Yet I focus on the complexity of human communication to emphasize a point: the importance of selecting *coauthors of worthiness.*

We have much to learn from our imperfections and little to gain by seeking perfection; indeed, I find that the best teachers are imperfect. I was blessed to find mentors who were pioneers in their disciplines worldwide, people who courageously defied those scientists who believed they had a monopoly on wisdom. These mentors chose to pay the price (academic disdain) of going beyond the pale in their respective professions. What I most admired about them were the elegance of their humility, their willingness to coauthor worthiness, and the wisdom they extracted from their imperfections. I strive to be just such an imperfect teacher.

LEARNING FROM IMPERFECT TEACHERS

One of the best ways to find imperfect teachers is straightforward: avoid those who believe they are perfect. So now let's debunk perfection and the merchants of platitudes.

Beware of Gurus Who . . .

. . . tell you to find stillness. Nothing, from the chains of amino acids to the present-moment experience of mindfulness, is ever still. Movement *is* life: the embodiment of perception and confirmation that you are in synchrony with all that exists and transcends. Unless you're dead, even your deepest serenity has movement. Rather than embrace the illusion of stillness, explore the movement of discovery.

It was tribal control of wonderment that turned an "abundance of curiosity" into "attention deficit disorder."

Health gurus *medicalize* living conditions they fail to understand, and medicalizing is a form of hegemony. In anthropology, hegemony means domination of one culture over another, with such insidious power that the dominated fail to see the dominators' impositions.

. . . tell you to give up your ego. Ego is the cultural self you need in order to participate in, contribute to, and learn from your world. To retreat to a cave for life while others suffer is to trade your contributions to the world for a life of spiritual selfishness. Of course, withdrawing from your world is your option, but not one I recommend. You should especially question the coherence of gurus with titles such as "venerable," "exalted," "revered," and other superlatives who instruct *you* to give up *your* ego.

. . . tell you being mindful is to be passively present. Mindfulness is an engagement with the present to explore the new and to detect mistakes. One of imperfection's lessons is to recognize that perfection implies no new learning. Can you imagine how boring you would be if you were perfect? There is much misunderstanding about the practice of mindfulness. In fact, calling mindfulness a "practice" is like saying "I am going to practice being alive." Meditation and other contemplative methods are some of the paths to mindfulness. In the applications section at the end of this chapter, I'll show you other ways to experience mindfulness.

. . . tell you to be one with the universe. Asking you to be one with anything other than yourself assumes you can be separated from your own existence. And although there is merit in metaphorically *seeing* union with the universe, it is more productive to *sense* your belongingness in this union. You don't have to be a tree to participate in the ecology of a forest. You learn the finite to speculate on the infinite. Find your world before you get lost in metaphors.

. . . tell you they are enlightened, or who entice you to believe that their spiritual narcissism is humility. We all have wisdom to gain from our imperfections, and little to offer from our delusions of grandeur. I once asked an "enlightened" guru how he experienced compassion. Without skipping a mystical beat, he answered, "I am beyond compassion." I showed him my compassion by leaving without telling him he was full of metaphysical manure. I respect bodhichittas and bodhisattvas because they are disciples of imperfection and compassion who try to help others on their own way to Buddhahood. I also respect seekers who, in Chögyam Trungpa's words, "cut through spiritual materialism." Trungpa was a Tibetan Buddhist master who wrote and taught on the topic of how to avoid spiritual narcissism. When my Tibetan lama teacher gave me a parchment signifying the lotus of wisdom, I asked him if his gift was recognition of my wisdom. He smiled and said, "It is for you to recognize how far you are from wisdom." All my mentors had great ways of bringing my ego back down to earth. I am pleased to inform you that I am still far from wisdom.

. . . entice you with winds of hope that cannot be harnessed. The responsibility of a teacher is to provide you with practical tools rather than platitudes. What is the use of wisdom that vanishes when you apply it to dissipating your fears and refining your love? While there is little benefit in spoon-feeding you instructions for every step of your explorations, it is equally impractical to leave you entirely with poetics when you need substance.

FOUR ATTRIBUTES FOR NAVIGATING TURBULENCE

Knowing what to avoid helps you clarify what you want. So why seek imperfection? Because you will gain more wisdom in the process of reaching for your goal than in attaining it. There are psychological benefits to be gained by exploring and learning the wisdom of imperfection: the *resilience* to transcend your disillusionments, the *perseverance* to overcome your obstacles, the *creativity* to find alternative solutions, and the *flexibility* to navigate turbulence. You may recall from chapter 5 that I found these four navigational tools in nearly every healthy centenarian I studied in different cultures on five continents. Interestingly, when we engage these four attributes of longevity in pursuit of our worthy goals, the joyful accomplishment we feel when we succeed derives from the satisfaction of mastering these attributes along the way. You can dance imperfectly around perfection without letting it seduce you into believing it exists.

In addition to celebrating mastery of the four attributes and accomplishing your goals, you can also celebrate with the coauthors of worthiness who grace your journey. For truly, nothing happens without coauthorship. And since you may not initially be aware of the coauthors who indirectly supported your worthiness during your journey, you will reap additional benefits if you acknowledge these subtle facilitators and share your accomplishments with them. Your gratitude attains a kind of elegance when you recognize that success never happens in a vacuum. And you refine the attributes of resilience, perseverance, creativity, and flexibility when you coauthor worthiness.

Your sense of self-worth is the stamp of approval for your journey toward abundance. But imagine how quickly those four positive attributes can turn into your worst obstacles if you lack tribal support. Your resilience is seen as arrogance, your perseverance as masochism, your creativity as naiveté, and your flexibility as weakness. Tribal control turns empowerment into helplessness when you defy the odds that should only be overcome within the pale. You anger the tribal gods when you take on challenges without their blessing, and they punish your transgressions by attacking your self-worth and self-confidence.

If you think I am being too harsh in my critique of tribal collectivism, scan your memory and recall circumstances in which your cultural editors expressed more support when you failed within the pale than when you succeeded beyond it. For example, a parent helping you rationalize poor academic performance while you were living at home and ignoring you when you excelled after you left for college. I am exposing these dynamics of forced tribal power to increase your awareness of why you may not value yourself as much as you are truly worth. *And* when you find the culprits who contributed to this state, I invite you to celebrate your discovery rather than place blame. Let go of your coauthors of known misery by disempowering the pain they caused you. Celebrating your liberation from disapproval is another lesson from *imperfection wisdom.*

YOUR THOUGHTS OF PERFECTION
AND YOUR IMPERFECT ACTIONS

When you think of what you want, you usually imagine an idealized scenario of achieving it, not the obstacles you will find when you move from thought into action. Even if you do ponder the obstacles, they seldom match the vicissitudes you will actually encounter on your way to your goal.

We plan our goals in the present and project them into a future about which we can only speculate. Then, all too often, we are disappointed when our perfect thoughts collide with an imperfect world. The circularity I am describing here is nothing new to you; we all know that dreams seldom match reality. What you may not know is that, if you learn to navigate imperfection, you can turn your disappointments into discovery. More important, if you navigate with *imperfection as your guide,* the obstacles you encounter on your journey can actually become shortcuts to your goals.

As you know by now, biocognition thrives on complexity, paradox, and subtleties of counterintuitive reasoning. An example is that if you learn *from* imperfection, you will increase your competence, but if you learn *with* imperfection you will increase your wisdom. Now let's bring these poetics into practice.

Wisdom in Your Imperfection

Learning from imperfection means extracting wisdom from your mistakes, and such lessons have positive aspects. But the common concept of a mistake is that it implies you're imperfect, and that learning from your mistakes brings you closer to perfection. In other words, you become *less* imperfect. Instead, I invite you to become *more* imperfect. Why? Am I entering the world of platitudes that I caution against? No, I am not. Instead, I am asking you to recontextualize the notion of *learning from the mistakes* that result from your imperfection into *learning with approximations* you make to glean wisdom from your imperfection. Every approximation you master to reach a goal becomes a goal. Gradually, as you continue to reach approximations, you experience a step-by-step mastery rather than falling short of your goal each time you try. What do I mean by approximations? Let's say that one day you want to run ten miles, but you are able to only run nine. You did not reach your goal of perfection, you reached something approximating it. The liberating way to view this is that you mastered and gained wisdom from an imperfect nine, not that you failed to reach a perfect ten.

In the first instance, your mistakes are errors you make because you are *flawed*. In the second instance, mistakes are not errors at all; they become approximations because you are wise. When you avoid making mistakes and learning from them as you pursue your goals, you reduce the instances in which you are faced with the flaws of your imperfection. But when you experience approximations and learn from them along the way, you increase your wisdom of imperfection.

Let me continue to clarify this paradoxical concept so you don't conclude that this proposal is simply a play on words. I am not replacing the word *mistake* with the word *approximation*. I would be giving you winds of hope that cannot be harnessed. Instead, I delineate the difference in contextual meaning between a *mistake caused by imperfection* and *approximation to the wisdom of imperfection*.

The context of a mistake includes its author, its coauthors, and the circumstances related to the mistake. Since we interpret causality based on context, in mistake context we designate the author, coauthors, or circumstances in order to determine why the mistake was made. Then we interpret the effects of a mistake based on where we place the blame. If you make a serious mistake at work when calculating the annual budget, your boss blames you and fires you. You are the cause, and the effect is to lose your job. But if the cause of the mistake is attributed to faulty computer hardware, the effect changes from firing you to repairing or replacing the computer; you keep your job and you may end up with a new laptop. In the first example, learning from the mistake may mean paying more attention to detail when calculating future budgets, and other preventive measures. In the second example, learning from the mistake may mean arranging for better computer maintenance—another preventive measure. Thus we can conclude that the learning-from-mistake context is designed to prevent imperfection.

Now let's apply the same situation within the context of learning from imperfection wisdom. Here, the purpose is to extract wisdom from your imperfection, or the imperfect conditions you face, rather than to focus on prevention, which is *indirectly achieved* when you find wisdom in your imperfection. The wisdom-in-imperfection context adds insights beyond prevention, and what's more, it engages synchronicity. I will offer examples further along to show you how synchronicity relates to finding wisdom in imperfection, as well as why I chose the term *approximation* to describe how you can optimize what you learn from imperfection. Although this new way of conceptualizing achievement may be difficult to assimilate, as you practice it, you will understand it beyond language. You will experience the felt meaning of mastering approximations.

While the implicit assumption in mistake context is *I make mistakes because I am imperfect,* the implicit assumption for wisdom-in-imperfection context is *mistakes are doorways to the wisdom of my imperfection.* In mistake context, cause equals blame and effect leads to prevention. In wisdom-of-imperfection context, cause equals a portal to a field and effect leads to wisdom.

Now let's apply the wisdom-of-imperfection context to the example of being fired because you made a mistake in calculating the annual budget. Since your mistake is now a portal, and the effect of the mistake leads to wisdom, here is what could happen: You enter the portal and begin to look for wisdom. You see that you despise your boss, that your commute to work is stressful, and that you have been considering working for yourself from home. As you confirm what you already know in your heart, your mind is now free to explore possible ways you can attain greater freedom. Your boss has still fired you, but now you feel gratitude for taking the step of coauthoring your freedom and for allowing synchronicity to find you.

Synchronicity can be defined as coincidental coherence that supports your actions by presenting conditions of timely significance. For example, the week before you were fired, your friend asked you if would consider doing financial consulting for his company. Your daughter wanted to know why you never go to her soccer games. Your boss called you frequently when you were on a recent vacation with your family.

If you give your imperfection wisdom time to unfold, the magnitude of the lessons you receive will astound and humble you, and you will experience unexpected joy. More important, you will confirm that you are not some sort of Darwinian accident living in a world of meaningless existence. But you must move faithfully forward with your joyful plans in order for synchronicity to grace you with auspicious meaning and impeccable timing.

Let me share my personal experience in applying what I am asking you to consider. Some years ago, I was very happily working for a state-of-the-art mindbody clinic at a world-class medical center. There, we were using my mindbody model to treat autoimmune illnesses. Patients came to the center from many countries because of the therapeutic success we were achieving by combining psychoneuroimmunology principles with insights from cultural anthropology—the effects of cultural beliefs on biology. Everything was working beautifully until our CEO, a humanist, was replaced by an executive who viewed hospitals as profit centers not unlike fast-food operations—a predatory stance, not a healing one. The new CEO concluded that other units were more profitable than our clinic. Thus, in his mind, it was a *mistake* to continue investing in the operation of our clinic. Since mistake context leads to prevention, our entire team was fired (two weeks before Christmas, no less) to prevent "revenue drain."

Was I blissful when I heard the news? Hell, no! In fact, I said something very sarcastic to deal with my disillusionment, "What a great Christmas gift." What I didn't know at the time was that this remark was a portal of approximation to imperfection wisdom. I realized later that the "gift" that holiday season was being fired. It led me into private practice, teaching seminars, and writing scientific articles. I had always wanted to do these things, but my job did not permit it. The firing was an approximation to my goal.

I think the most significant part of this story is how and when I realized the auspicious meaning of the word "gift." After allowing myself to experience the embodiment and displacement of my initial anger and fear (using the techniques I share in this book), I went to my favorite Indian restaurant to celebrate my unemployment without knowing the meaning of my celebration. It was a *feedforward* event, a condition in the present with meaning that unfolds in the future. When I was finishing my meal, a waiter who knew me well asked me, "How's the job?" At that instant, an epiphany unfolded before my eyes when I responded without thinking, "Tonight, I am celebrating my decision to go into private practice!"

My sarcastic remark when I was fired expressed what I call a *soon-to-unfold event*, and my celebration afterward permitted synchronicity to unveil its meaning. And my familiar waiter, who had never asked me about my job until that moment, became a coauthor of my synchronicity.

I use this story to illustrate the approximation-to-imperfection wisdom context I have described, and also so I can offer you the moral it contains. When you're first hit with disturbing news, avoid the extremes of Pollyannaish optimism and victimhood, and engage the four attributes to navigate turbulence—resilience, perseverance, creativity, and flexibility. Pollyanna merely glosses over her pain, and victims can never even recognize the portals of imperfection wisdom.

APPROXIMATION PORTALS

Here in the tenth chapter, I am pleased to be able to get into greater depth in conveying the lessons of biocognitive consciousness. You have become more fluent in the language, and the more familiar you become, the more joy you will find in your biocognitive journey.

The approximation concept I am introducing in this chapter is both complex and liberating. Understanding *biocognitive approximation* opens a doorway to your innate wisdom—in this case, the wisdom of your imperfection.

I will clarify the biocognitive concept of approximation by first explaining its meaning in complexity theory. *Approximation algorithm* is the technical term I borrowed from complexity theory and modified to explain how we can approach what we cannot completely reach. An algorithm is a step-by-step procedure to make a calculation, a set of instructions to reach a solution. Combined, the two words mean "instructions to approximate solutions."

Why only approximate? Because some complexity problems in mathematics cannot be completely solved. The best we can do is *approximate* to arrive at optimal solutions. But since to solve is to know, we can apply the concept of approximation to complex psychological conditions that cannot be completely known.

Now let's bring complexity theory to biocognition. Just as we can never reach perfection, we cannot completely know imperfection. I argue that to ensure that our learning never stops, our brain was designed to function in what I call *relational incompleteness*. In order to learn, you have to *relate* what you want to know. You have to relate maleness with femaleness to know your gender; tallness with shortness to know your height. But most concepts you want to know cannot be known completely. The wisdom of imperfection is a complex concept we can approximate but never completely know.

You can celebrate the complexity of your brain when you recognize the beauty of relational incompleteness. Imagine your friends' reactions if you said, "Let's have dinner tonight to celebrate the relational incompleteness of our brains." Remember, you have to give your coauthors time to catch up with your joy of discovery.

DISTRACTIONS FROM YOUR WORTHINESS

Now let's ask some challenging questions to take this contextual theory of imperfection wisdom to its logical conclusion. If mistake leads to prevention, approximation leads to imperfection wisdom, and both contexts reduce the frequency of our errors, what context reduces our worthiness? Also, do we reduce our worthiness by mistake or on purpose? Since we know that self-sabotage reduces our worthiness, is self-sabotage a mistake or a deliberate action on our part?

Before you are aware of self-destructive behavior, it is mistake. The instant you recognize it, it ceases to be mistake. I argue that self-sabotage is *purposeful mindlessness,* determined action without awareness of intention. For example, the purposeful mindlessness of self-sabotage can help us understand why addictions and other self-distractive behaviors are difficult to change by appealing to logic. Yes, you read that correctly. *Self-distractive* is a biocognitive term I use to define *destructive distractions.* Later in the chapter, I will explain the difference between mindlessness and mindfulness.

If addictive behavior is a mistake, all we need to do is correct what was mistaken. Try telling a cocaine addict to stop using because cocaine is dangerous, and you will see that substance abuse is purposeful behavior. Now here comes the most challenging question: is the cause of addiction disease or purposeful action? I believe that addictions are sociocultural self-distractions that serve to avoid worthiness, and are not disease at all. Is this naive theorizing? After treating several thousand addicts, I don't think so. If you assume that addiction is a disease, you can't attribute any purposeful action on your part to something that simply "happens" to you. In other words, you can't will yourself into disease. Of course, some destructive behavior can lead to disease, but if your diagnosis is "addiction," your "disease" status frees you from authorship; you are responsible for your substance abuse only until your behavior is diagnosed. From that moment on, the cause of your behavior shifts from your purposeful action to your inevitable genetics. You are given medical permission to be *diseased* without hope of a cure. Do you see how tribal control shifts your dependence from substance abuse to *within-the-pale medicine?* In the practical section toward the end of this chapter, I will teach you how to effectively change self-distractive behavior.

This argument involves more than addictions. The concept of self-distraction also applies to obsessions, compulsions, and any other excessive behavior. I chose addiction as an example because it is the most difficult to treat and the most misunderstood of self-distractive behaviors.

THE IMPERFECTION PARADOX

Why do I propose that addictions, obsessions, and compulsions are sociocultural self-distractions to avoid worthiness? First, consider the correct clinical meanings of addiction, obsession, and compulsion.

Addiction is the *acquired dependence* on a psychoactive substance and requires replenishment when blood levels of that substance drop. The drop in blood level causes withdrawal symptoms that are responsible for the vicious cycle that maintains addiction. Obsessions are intrusive *thoughts* that are difficult to stop. Compulsions are intrusive *actions* that are difficult to stop. Eating disorders, inordinate sexuality, gambling, and other excessive, uncontrollable behaviors are compulsions, not addictions. Uncontrollable thoughts about sex, the Internet, and any other intrusive thinking are obsessions, not addictions or compulsions. Uncontrollable use of cocaine, alcohol, and other psychoactive drugs are addictions, not compulsions or obsessions.

Don't be too concerned if you have been using these terms interchangeably; many health care professionals make the same mistake. But now, since you know better, you can cease to "abuse" these three terms.

Addictions, obsessions, and compulsions are distractions from self-worthiness, and are *not* disease. But I want to emphatically clarify that although these excessive dysfunctional behaviors are not diseases, they require professional help and should not be taken lightly. It is also imperative to understand that the function of these excessive behaviors is to distract you from self-worthiness, not to masochistically hurt yourself. Independent of purpose, self-sabotaging distractions can cause considerable mindbody damage.

With these concepts now established, I can introduce the *imperfection paradox* to help you understand the illusive nature of perfection. Most of us would like to be perfect. Competition to achieve excellence starts early in life. What may appear as lack of ambition is actually helplessness resulting from repeated failure to achieve perfection. Now, you can recognize that perfection is elusive and choose to redirect your pursuit of it, or you can continue the quixotic chase of the windmills of perfection. If you equate your worthiness with perfection, you will be compelled to measure your achievements against illusory standards—and here is where the imperfection paradox comes in.

Addictions, compulsions, and obsessions are distractions to maintain consistency with the false premise that perfection is attainable, but only for others. Self-sabotage based on this faulty logic has two functions: to punish you because you are flawed and to avoid evidence that you are not flawed. Success becomes your worst enemy. Paradoxically, you choose unwanted imperfection to avoid the perfection you yearn for.

WHAT IS MINDFULNESS?

Mindfulness is a term that has gained significant popularity in the self-help market, and unfortunately, anything marketed runs the risk of being misunderstood, simplistically packaged, and misappropriated. Mindfulness is usually sold as something special, esoteric, and difficult to achieve without extensive instructions. There is nothing wrong with selling instructions as long as they are accurate and demystified. You will hear that to be mindful is to be completely present while observing without judgment in a meditative state of calm. You will also hear that mindfulness means disengaging from automatic behavior and shifting to consciously being in the present.

Remarkably, although these descriptions of mindfulness are mostly accurate, you will find little information in the self-help market about *mindlessness*—the diametric opposite of mindfulness. Why is it important to know the opposite of what you are trying to learn? Because, since most of us spend 99 percent of our time in mindlessness, when we *are* asked to learn about mindfulness, we are being asked to learn something we rarely do, without exploring the function of what we *constantly* do.

Let's understand the function of mindlessness before we delve into the wisdom of mindfulness. The apophatic method you learned in chapter 9 will be helpful here. This method of inquiry reaches understanding by negation, a roundabout way of knowing a boundless concept by describing what the concept is *not*. For example, in apophatic theology, God is not man; God is not a person. In poetics, love is not possession, and love is not need. Both examples lead to meaning by default. The apophatic method allows *approximation meaning* of concepts that are beyond complete knowing; you intuit meaning by describing what it is not instead of defining what it is. Just as approximation meaning helped you understand perfection, it will also help you understand another illusive concept I will now introduce: control.

So what is mindlessness? Here are some examples of mindlessness behaviors: when you cough from smoking a cigarette and you continue to smoke between coughs; when you repeatedly press an elevator button to make it arrive faster; when you are in a loud restaurant and you shout to be heard without recognizing your own intrusive noise; when you are stuck in traffic and continually honk your horn to make other vehicles move; when you scream at your children to teach them not to scream; when you drive to your destination and arrive without awareness of how you got there.

I can go on indefinitely, but you get the picture. Notice that each example shows mindlessness distraction. What is the function of this? Why do we engage our foolishness rather than embody our imperfection wisdom? Because we are trying to control the uncontrollable. We are not aware we are distracting ourselves and *mistakenly* assuming we have control. Just as we seek perfection, we also seek control. Both perfection and control are conditions we can only approximate by understanding their boundlessness and illusiveness. Mindlessness is being unaware of our distractions and our flawed solutions. By living in our mindlessness world, we avoid mindful recognition of our lack of control.

But let's dig deeper into the functions of mindlessness. In the examples I just related, you can clearly see a smoker avoiding awareness of self-damage; helpless attempts to control traffic, an elevator, and an intrusive noise; and a parent teaching "do as I say, not as I do." But what are you trying to control when you drive mindlessly to your destination? This last example explains another component of mindlessness: not being in the present. Mindlessness driving exemplifies a focus on the past or future. In other words, when you are *thinking* about something rather than *being* present, you are either recalling the past or anticipating the future. Your brain is so adaptive that it can pursue your objective even when you tune your objective entirely out of your awareness. Unfortunately, we abuse this developmental marvel by spending too much time on automatic pilot.

Now you know that mindlessness equals not being in the present, and that its functions are to avoid awareness of your flawed solutions and your lack of control. More important, you have indirectly learned about mindfulness by exploring mindlessness. The apophatic lesson is this: if mindlessness is what mindfulness is not, then mindfulness is being in the present to discover novelty and mistakes. When you are *present* in the present, not *absent* in the present, you are aware of what is new around you and of the ways in which you are distracting yourself with flawed solutions to avoid your lack of control.

Notice, I applied a modified version of the classical apophatic method here. Instead of strictly describing what mindfulness is *not*, I used mindlessness to identify the diametric opposite of what mindfulness *is*. Why not simply describe mindfulness directly? Because, since mindfulness is a boundless experience, you can only approximate its meaning. As you learn mindfulness, you will continue to intuit additional meaning from its boundless totality.

FROM THEORY TO PRACTICE

The new concepts I have introduced in this chapter can be powerful agents of change if you learn how to apply them to your challenges. I will now give you practical tools to work with these concepts in the order in which I presented them. You can apply each tool using the contemplative methods you have learned in other chapters, or simply by sitting in a quiet place where you can experience the conditions I will ask you to explore. Also, you can apply the tools interchangeably, depending on your challenges. For example, methods for recontextualizing cause and effect, changing self-distractive behavior, and experiencing mindfulness are different ways to approach a challenge. As you learn to apply these tools, you will discover how to maximize their effectiveness in different contexts. You can practice using the tools based on the challenges you want to confront, and you can prudently decide the frequency and intensity of your practice.

How to Recontextualize the Cause
and Effect of Your Challenges

Select a recurring problem in your personal or professional life that you wish to change, for example, habitual tardiness or an inability to save money.

❖ Identify the cause to which you assign the problem and the solution you choose; for example, you can't save money because your parents never could (a learned cause).

❖ Identify the cultural editor who taught you to arrive at the cause you attributed to the problem. This may require some digging, because you are not used to looking at a cause as something you learned. You can also learn to attribute cause from personal experience without a cultural editor's involvement, but there is always a cultural context.

❖ When you identify the cause, determine whether you learned it within the pale or beyond the pale. Did the problem happen while you were complying with tribal rules or defying them?

❖ Experience how you embody the memory of the cause and the solution you learned. Breathe slowly and allow the physical manifestation to dissipate before continuing.

❖ Find an alternative cause and solution for your problem from a framework of worthiness. View mistakes as windows to your imperfection wisdom. If you attributed a mistake to your cause and found a solution to prevent your mistake, look for wisdom in the imperfection of your mistake and your solution. For example, you find that you can't save money because you live beyond your means—a way to live up to what you learned from your parents. You can readjust your overspending lifestyle and release the dysfunctional lesson.

❖ Identify the wisdom you extracted from your mistake and your solution, and experience how the new context manifests in your mindbody.

❖ Commit to attributing a worthy cause and solution to all recurring problems.

❖ If you identify coauthors in future recurring problems, give your coauthor(s) permission to not like your new worthiness response. Coauthors may not be ready to evolve with you.

❖ If you forget to implement your new strategy when you confront a future problem, celebrate the discovery rather than punish yourself for forgetting. Being patient with your imperfection requires self-compassion.

❖ Look for hidden benefits in your old cause and solution. How did you control others with your dysfunctional distractions? For example, you conveniently "forgot" to bring your wallet to a restaurant, and for the second time, your friend pays for your dinner.

❖ Commit to giving up the benefits of unworthy designation of cause and effect. Celebrate the worthiness gained from giving up your helplessness and relentless pursuit of control.

How to Change Your Self-Distractive Behavior

If you are dealing with addiction, obsession, or compulsion disorders, consult a health care professional to help you enhance what you will learn in this section. If he or she does not agree with my concept of learned sociocultural dysfunction, you can still benefit from focusing on your distractions from worthiness and from slowly facing your fear of not being perfect or in complete control. Also, you may find qualified health care professionals who are willing to consider this model of mindbody culture.

❖ Find a recurrent self-distraction you use to avoid mistakes, out-of-control anxiety, or any other self-distractive behavior that alienates you from your worthiness. For example, eating or smoking to reduce anxiety, or lying to hide mistakes.

❖ When you identify your self-distracting pattern, experience how it manifests in your mindbody. Breathe calmly. Notice that your inner turbulence dissipates faster when you observe rather than attempt to control your experience.

❖ Identify helplessness in your self-distractive pattern and ways in which you may be punishing yourself. For example, excessive alcohol consumption to avoid confronting a dysfunctional marriage and attributing the drinking problem to your genes.

❖ Celebrate your discovery of how your self-distraction robs you of your worthiness. Celebration can range from enjoying your immediate experience of triumph to identifying something worthy you can do for yourself at a later date.

❖ Redefine self-distractions as mistaken signals, and identify your correct action. For example, if you have an eating disorder, you may be confusing signals of anxiety, boredom, shame, or any other turbulence with signals of hunger. In this case, you mistook your inner commotion for hunger.

❖ Identify what you would have to give up and confront if you replace your self-distraction with correct action. For example, if you learn you are eating when you are anxious, you will have to give up food as your anti-anxiety solution and confront what makes you anxious.

❖ Imagine you are six months into the future and you are no longer using your self-distractive pattern. In that scenario of worthiness, what relationships do you have to modify, and how do you fill the vacuum left when you gave up your self-distraction? Remember, although self-distractions are dysfunctional, they have a significant place in your life. Be aware that releasing known misery causes anxiety.

❖ Enter the discomfort caused by the vacuum and experience how it manifests in your mindbody.

❖ Breathe slowly and observe your turbulence as waves disappearing on the shore. Avoidance increases turbulence. Observation reduces turbulence.

❖ Experience how turbulence diminishes with each exhalation. In the metaphor of turbulence as waves, your exhalation is the shore dissipating the waves.

❖ Apply the tools you learned here as much as you need to. Be prudent and patient. You have a lifetime to joyfully discover wisdom in your imperfection.

How to Experience Your Mindfulness

Now you know that mindfulness does not have to involve deep meditation. In fact, some contemplative methods impede mindfulness because they do not allow you to be consciously present. I recognize that some practitioners may disagree with my concept of mindfulness as active engagement with your present, but in my view, they confuse the state of mindfulness with the state of deep contemplative consciousness.

❖ Sit comfortably in a quiet place and observe for a few minutes what you're experiencing in your mindbody. You can do this exercise with your eyes open or closed.

❖ Identify repetitive cycles in your observations. For example, are you noticing repeating cycles going from awareness of one part of your body to another part you have already experienced, or from one thought to another thought you have already had? Recognizing repetitive cycles of awareness is discovery. Any discovery is mindfulness.

❖ In addition to discovering repetitive cycles, look for novelty as you observe your mindbody experience. What do you notice that is new? For example, did you notice new thoughts or emotions in your stream of consciousness?

❖ If you closed your eyes to experience your mindbody world, open your eyes and begin to experience your surroundings that way.

❖ Discover repetitive cycles. For example, looking at a wall, then looking at a window and returning to the same wall. You are in mindfulness the moment you discover you're in reruns.

❖ Break repetitive cycles and mindless scanning by discovering novelty in your observations. For example, you may notice a bird fly to your window. The paint on the wall is lighter than you thought. The window has six panes, not four. You notice that where you are sitting is not as comfortable as you initially thought it would be. Discovering new information and mistakes, by being present, is mindfulness.

❖ Purposely look for anything new in your mindbody and external observations.

❖ Notice how discovering things you had not noticed before, as well as mistakes, takes on a new felt meaning.

❖ Enjoy the intellectual, physical, and emotional effects of discovering novelty and mistakes.

❖ After you complete the exercises in this section, commit to looking for discoveries in your daily routines and celebrating whenever you catch your mistakes. To be mindful is to be fully engaged in your present.

Congratulations! If you followed these instructions, you have just entered mindfulness without having to seek a master in Nepal. These biocognitive methods, like many others you have learned in this book, are deceptively simple because you don't have to jump any complicated hurdles to experience the power they have to change your world. But the elegance of their simplicity shines only when you apply them mindfully to the challenges in your life.

You can practice the exercises in the sequence presented here or choose to apply them based on whatever challenges emerge in your life.

❖ ❖ ❖

Whenever you are ready, let's go on to chapter 11, where I will show you how to navigate chaos with uncertainty as your guide by entering portals of synchronicity.

Portals of Synchronicity

THE DRIFT

In biocognitive theory, I introduce a concept of coincidental experiences that I call the *drift:* portals to synchronistic pathways. These out-of-order states are undulations (ripple effects) of deeper meaning that you can access to transform your life from a mundane one to a life filled with celebrations of exalting discoveries. Instead of the usual esoteric interpretations of synchronicity, biocognitive theory asserts that the drift is a time/space of *interconnectedness* that anyone can access if they use the right tools of observation. In this chapter, I'll teach you how to observe what is already happening in these out-of-order portals, which are to be entered without any preconceived outcome in mind.

Some of the observational methods you will need include *feedforward, apophatic inquiry,* and *prolepsis.* These incidental learning methods will help to access the subtle ingredients of meaningful relationships and an abundance of health, wealth, and love. This may sound like an empty promise, but there is substance here. With this approach, I am not asking you to believe in what I am teaching you. Instead, I am offering you the tools to reclaim the personal power you were taught to disown.

Before exploring these methods, I'll share why I believe that understanding extraordinary events can help you find beneficial meaning in the things that happen in your life, both good and bad. We tend to conceptualize our good fortune using different tools from those we use for misfortune. This is understandable because we enjoy good things in life and avoid or endure what pains us. Both conditions have undulations of wisdom, but we tend to focus on enjoying the good and suffering through the bad. And although we know that lessons in life can come from both joy and misery, we don't realize that our interpretations of each condition determine our access to the wisdom in both.

Even in the best-case scenario, we fall short of what we can learn from *happenings* in our lives when we overlook the wisdom of uncertainty. For example, you feel blessed when good fortune comes your way, and "make the best" of your misfortune. Although these responses are commendable, they are both based on how your culture taught you to deal with life rather than what you can learn from *your own* life. Some of the cultural premises we learn include: life is good, life is suffering, deny pain, rationalize misfortunes, and so on. None, however, deals with the interconnected nature of events, and consequently these premises obscure how to navigate the uncertainty of events. By the way, uncertainty is embedded in both fortune and misfortune. More important, "out-of-order" does not mean "random."

Let's look at the drift from a scientific perspective to see how you can apply its principles to effectively navigate uncertainty in your life.

Interconnectedness

Out-of-order conditions seem random and meaningless. Yet this is a misconception that stems from popularizing scientific terms and giving them inaccurate definitions. For example, the mathematical definition of randomness is zero predictability. In fact, because true randomness is so difficult to achieve, when researchers "randomize" subjects to experimental and control groups, they use highly technical random number generators. Rather than the zero predictability of randomness, out-of-order events have complex interconnectedness with multiple out-of-sequence contributions from different origins. To further clarify the concept of out-of-order events, I'll quote Herodotus, a Greek historian of the fifth century BCE: "In times of peace, children bury their parents; war disrupts the order of nature, and parents bury their children."

Herodotus's powerful observation illustrates how war can disrupt the natural order of life and create a sense of meaninglessness and uncertainty.

But what may not be so clear is that, rather than being the result of a single cause, war is a portal of interconnectedness that leads to out-of-order events. So, for example, not all soldiers will die in battle, because war sets a stage for the unfolding of multiple events that could lead to dying, sustaining wounds, or surviving unscathed. While unpredictability causes uncertainty, disruption of natural order mimics randomness and precludes meaning.

I can tell you from a neuropsychological perspective that an out-of-order, life-threatening condition is the main cause of post-traumatic stress disorder. Why? Because the brain is designed to process the natural order of life, and when confronted with an out-of-order condition that is life-threatening, it compresses the traumatic experience to process it *after* the danger is over. But since recalling traumatic events produces anxiety, the person who had the experience avoids "processing" it, and the unresolved shock eventually causes sporadic panic attacks: the brain's desperate attempt to decompress the trauma.

Cultural Ingredients in Out-of-Order Events

As a serious student of biocognition, you should wonder how culture interacts with life-threatening, out-of-order events. I propose that it depends on how your cultural editors define the meaning of out-of-order events. Depending on your culture, their cause might be attributed to karma, destiny, divinity, luck, evil spirits, martyrdom, magic, and so on. Thus, cultural meaning brings order to disorder and the endurance to navigate uncertainty. For example, an out-of-order death attributed to the will of God is interpreted very differently from one attributed to chance.

Now that I've addressed negative out-of-order events, let's look at how they compare with their positive counterparts. I used war, the most infamous human invention, to illustrate the worst disruption of life's natural order. But what could I cite to illustrate the same degree of impact from positive, out-of-order events?

There's no equivalent to the value of human life, and there's no greater anguish than parents burying their children. Thus, rather than trying to juxtapose life and death, I'll choose love to illustrate what's involved in an out-of-order, joyful event. Let's say you're flying to Rio de Janeiro for a well-deserved vacation, but five hours into the flight, the plane's electrical system malfunctions, and the pilot decides to divert course and land in Belo Horizonte. You're annoyed to begin with, and to make things worse, the airline mechanics there are on strike; you're told you can either wait for a couple of days or take a bus to Rio.

You decide to rent a car and stop at the picturesque colonial town of Ouro Preto (Black Gold) because the name is familiar. You remember it from a novel you read in college. When you arrive, the town has a certain charm—beyond its eighteenth-century architecture—that entices you to stay for a couple of days. You're bewitched, and Rio has taken second place. That evening, you choose to dine at Contos de Reis (Tales of Kings), a cozy restaurant recommended by the innkeeper at the B&B where you're staying. When you're seated, you recognize a fellow passenger from your diverted flight who has been told that all the tables are taken. Impulsively, and happy to see a familiar face, you invite this person to join you for dinner.

The conversation is alluring. You order wine, and when you toast, your eyes meet. And in what feels like a time/space compression, this stranger transforms into someone you could love for the rest of your life. By the end of the evening, you have compared experiences and found a connection that defies all reason—and welcomes magic. You have found your partner for life!

Too good to be true? An improbable fantasy to entice you? I can assure you that something remarkably similar happened to me five years ago that resulted in my moving from the United States to Montevideo, Uruguay.

NAVIGATING UNCERTAINTY

Now I'll extract clues from segments of these two out-of-order examples to illustrate how portals of synchronicity unfold and how to navigate their interconnectedness. To help you conceptualize the ingredients of synchronicity, imagine a web of interwoven pathways that has no underlying order or design—at least none you can discern—something like haphazardly connected doodles representing roads. But suppose there is an underlying design, unknown to you. Now imagine drawing a straight line so you can travel on that web from point A, where you are now, to point B, your destination, without knowing the underlying design. You have superimposed a visual, linear, and orderly pathway on an invisible, nonlinear, disorderly web.

You begin your travel expecting that the order you imposed from point A to point B will get you from here to there because you believe the line you drew will hold true. Most of the time, the linear order will work, and you will reach your destination unaware of any underlying interconnectedness. Then one day, certain conditions *coemerge* from the hidden, disorderly web and your linearity from points A to B is blocked. Without recognizing that there are other pathways, you continue to assume your way is the only way. You keep pushing to confirm your reality and decrease your uncertainty.

By chance, the next time this happens, you take one of the detouring pathways, and since they all are interconnected, you find meaningful coincidences and experience synchronicity. The "meaningful" coincidences are always there to unfold when you follow the drift: you enter a portal of synchronicity. But there is a catch; since the portals are tentative and hidden from linear order, you can't seek them directly or at will. You must wait for an invitation to detour using a different navigational compass.

The Nonlinear Compass

I invite you to see a world that is interwoven with disordered pathways that become available to you when you shift navigational compasses. If you proceed without shifting compasses, it will be like trying to get around Chicago using a map of Seattle. There's no mystery here. I will clarify, once again, using neuropsychology.

Roughly, our brain has two perceptual modes. The left side of the brain makes sense of linear information using sequential tools. These include language, logical reasoning, arithmetic, and other nonspatial capacities. Conversely, the right side of the brain handles the nonlinear tasks: intuition, musical comprehension, higher math, and other information requiring visual-spatial mapping. I should note that I am grossly oversimplifying brain function. The brain is highly malleable, and the two hemispheres function with interwoven horizons rather than rigid frontiers. For example, to sing a song, you require the left hemisphere of your brain for the linear aspects of the lyrics, and the right hemisphere for the spatial arrangement and intonation of the music.

But after this quick neuropsychological detour, I want to emphasize that, to make sense of a highly complex world, our brain imposes linearity and sequence to navigate and decrease uncertainty in our daily tasks. Thus, the linearity component is necessary to perceive sequential order, but when we encounter out-of-sequence events, we must shift our compass from *confirmation* to *observation*. An out-of-order event is an invitation to a portal, and observation is what allows successful entrance. Once you're in, the synchronicity will enthrall you, and its complexity will humble you. But you won't know you have entered the portal until the synchronicity shakes you into recognizing that you are not a Darwinian accident void of meaning. Rather than aimless meandering, the drift is meaningful digression.

Now I'll use some *segments of meaning* from the two out-of-order examples to illustrate how the drift works. Your planned Rio vacation was detoured by the mechanical malfunctioning of your plane (the first out-of-order invitation to a portal). If, instead of considering the option of driving to Rio with a detour to Ouro Preto, you had insisted upon reaching your final destination, you would not have recognized the portal that led to finding the love of your life. The second out-of-order event (portal) was the fortuitous meeting at the restaurant that sparked your invitation to dine. You may have also noticed that synchronicity had already surfaced when you connected the name of the town, Ouro Preto, with the novel you read in college. Although navigating the drift does not guarantee fortunate results, at worst it adds novelty to your existence, and at best . . . opportunities for endless celebration.

Entangling Soon-to-Unfold Events

The plot thickens, but with the right tools, almost anything is possible. I am reminded of Archimedes's dare, "Give me a long enough lever and a fulcrum, and I shall move the earth." Fortunately, our objective here is less ambitious than that, but no less fascinating than knowing the drift.

We're all familiar with the term *feedback*. Although the technical definition comes from the science of acoustics, the popular description of feedback is well known: information from the past to guide your present. But here, I will introduce you to one of the tools to access the drift: *feedforward.* Just like its counterpart, the technical definition for feedforward comes from one of the branches of engineering, but in biocognition, I give it a special operational meaning. Before I define it, to help you make sense of the concept, recall the web of interwoven, disorderly pathways. Although you can superimpose a linear path on the web, there are underlying interconnections before and after your linear path. In terms of time, some are from the past, and others are waiting to unfold in the future. And although I am not suggesting time travel, the interconnectedness does not end because time passes. Thus, my definition for feedforward is this: an out-of-order event in the present, with unfolding meaning or relevance in the future; a component of interconnectedness and its synchronistic portals.

When you accept the interconnectedness component of synchronicity, feedforward can be an effective tool for accessing synchronicity. How? You can use feedforward to celebrate, in the present, a future event: an entangling, fortuitous, soon-to-unfold event. In other words, simply celebrate in the present without knowing the reason, and wait for the event to unfurl in the future. Because of what I have gleaned from personal experience and from teaching this method to many of my students, I invite you to try it and allow its process to coemerge.

Let me play devil's advocate and assume this is my delusion, and there is no such thing as feedforward. If you celebrate anyway, you will still benefit by not having to wait for a reason to have an enjoyable experience, and you will become a better observer of what facilitates your good fortune. The curiosity and wonderment this model of living provides has powerful psychoneuroimmunological benefits: curiosity improves memory and general brain function, and wonderment reduces pessimistic beliefs that support helplessness and trigger weak immunity. So, analogous to Pascal's wager about the existence of God, I invite you to consider feedforward as my *interconnectedness wager* and allow it to increase the quality of your life! My close friends and family practice this regularly and make delightful discoveries. Of course, be selective about whom you share feedforward celebrations with. Cynics and pessimists will deny its value to their graves because it might bring them joy—a dangerous emotion for those who lack self-love.

Apophatic Inquiry

I discussed and explained apophasis in chapter 9 as a contemplative method to negate distractions. Now I am going to teach you how to use apophatic inquiry to navigate uncertainty. Let's return to the example of war, and how it disrupts the natural order of life. Apophatic inquiry reaches noncontextual meaning through negation. Contextual meaning is not sufficient to enable parents who have to bury their children to find serenity. Apophasis can be an indirect path to interconnectedness as it can bring existential closure to circumstances in which logic cannot reach the heart.

Finding interconnectedness is another path to serenity. In the example of casualties of war, the apophatic negation process can include: a son does not die at war to defend his country, for the glory of God, because of bad luck, for heroism, by accident, from carelessness, and so on. When you exhaust the intellectual pursuit of meaning, you are left in a linguistic void of reasoning, logic, orderly sequence, and any other categorizing. More important, this noncontextual vacuum is also free of uncertainty. Why? Because uncertainty is fed by a need to know, to reinstate order, and to regain control. But when apophasis turns off the intellectual vehicle that feeds the vicious cycle of having to know, it removes the linearity that blocks access to portals of interconnectedness. I've witnessed patients who have had to bury their children find serenity they could only describe as, "We are not alone."

Prolepsis

Prolepsis is a very enigmatic term from the Greek, defined as a preconception, the anachronistic representation of something existing before its proper or historical time. Let me clarify its meaning and application to interconnectedness by using concrete examples.

Approximately 3,800 years ago, the Maya made wheels for several reasons: as toys, to keep time, and to chart their astrology. But they never made the leap to build wheels for transportation: they existed before the proper time to discover their main function. Leonardo da Vinci sketched a helicopter-like machine that had to wait five hundred years before it could be made to fly. Several of Einstein's discoveries existed before their time, waiting for the invention of instruments to confirm his contributions to physics.

Prolepsis can be another tool to access the interconnected web of nonlinear space. As I do in each chapter, toward the end of this one, I'll teach you how to use these tools. But for now, let's look at how prolepsis relates to interconnectedness. I can give you an example from the corporate world. Although I didn't mentor Steve Jobs, my use of prolepsis has some similarity to his *reality distortion field.* He met with his engineers at Apple, and when they said his idea for improving a product was not possible, he retorted, "Yes, it is possible, and you can do it." Eventually, they entered his reality distortion field and *invented* what he envisioned. The iPad, iPhone, and other Apple products existed in Steve's mind before their historical time.

So how do you harness prolepsis? I'll give you some examples of how I use it in clinical and corporate environments. I have patients imagine they are living in the year 3050, and a cure for their illness was found many years back. I ask them to visualize that their illness was as challenging as polio was before Salk discovered the vaccine in 1952, and that their disease, too, has been successfully eradicated. (In fact, when Salk was working on his vaccine, he imagined he was a virus, in order to help him decipher how polio behaved in different environments.) Prolepsis is a tool to access what physicist David Bohn called the *implicate order,* unharnessed wisdom with potential to surface before its historical time.

Although most of my patients with unsolved diseases do not find cures for them by using prolepsis, it empowers them to embrace hope and not feed their sense of helplessness. On the more substantive side, I've developed effective treatments for fibromyalgia, obesity, and addictions using some of the tools I am introducing in this chapter. And in the corporate mentoring I do for Fortune 100 executives, I've applied prolepsis and other biocognitive tools to create revolutionary incentive options, discover new markets, and improve the personal health of executives who work under relentless pressure.

ENGAGING THE DRIFT

From a practical perspective, the drift is a process in which outcome cannot be predicted from segment to segment because our senses and the instruments of science are not able to chart simultaneity. If we dare to approach uncharted territory, we need to proceed with faith in a fortuitous outcome. Science requires evidence in order to believe, whereas faith requires belief without evidence. But I'll remind you, I am not referring to religious and spiritual faith. This is more about recognizing interconnectedness than looking for cause and effect. You can look for cause and correlation of what you experience, and your choice will mostly depend on the level of certainty that makes you comfortable.

For example, when you have a headache, you take analgesics to relieve the pain because you are comfortable with assigning the cause to tension. But if you go deeper into the chain of causes, you might find the tension was triggered by your boss's negative response to your performance at work; going deeper, you find your boss reminds you of how your father mistreated you; and even deeper, how his father mistreated him; and so on, without end. Indeed, even the most exact sciences rely on this principle of cause determined by comfort level. Nothing can be unquestionably proven—the best we can do in science is agree on the statistical probability we are willing to accept to indicate that our results are not based on chance. So you see? Scientists place their faith in statistical probability, and not in irrefutable causes. Although I have faith in science, I want to assure you that science does not have a monopoly on truth.

On the other hand, correlation means association with what appears related to an experience or observation. Some correlations are valid and some are not. For example, if you drink a Pepsi and wear a green shirt when your headache starts, although the soft drink and your shirt could be associated with your headache, you will most likely conclude the two items are not contributing to the cause. Thus, you can find causal and noncausal correlations in any experience.

Finding versus Discovering

If you look for the cause of what you experience, when you *find* it, your faith in the cause will grow. Conversely, if you *discover* the unfolding of what you experience, your faith in interconnectedness will grow. Hence, you can look either for single cause-and-effect or for simultaneity.

To engage the drift, you must suspend predictability so you can discover interconnectedness. You will recognize the portals when you're already in the drift. Finding and discovering have different cognitive registries. Finding requires searching for a known outcome, whereas discovering involves observing the unfolding of events that gain meaning *after* you experience them. When you're discovering, you don't know what you're seeking until it unfolds.

After you enter a portal of synchronicity, occurrences that initially appeared improbable and without connection become meaningful in a multidimensional way. We are so unaccustomed to the drift that when we encounter its inherent simultaneity, we view it as a highly improbable but meaningful coincidence. Yet in the drift, synchronicity is a frequent occurrence readily available to you in the discovery mode. The aphorism "seek and you shall find" does not work well with the drift because its portals are out-of-order conditions that must be interpreted as opportunities to discover, not obstacles in your journey.

Indeterminate Locality

Understanding the concept and language of the drift prepares you to identify its portals and navigate its pathways. And although it's analogous to entering a new dimension, when you apply the proper tools, the drift is as tangible as any other experience in your life. But I don't want to leave you with the impression that the drift is another way of saying "go with the flow." In fact, when you confront turbulence, it might be unwise to "flow" because you could enter without the proper tools to handle a potentially dangerous condition.

So what's the difference? The drift does not mean giving in to obstructions on your journey and taking whatever comes. It actually involves several conscious steps. Thus, rather than flowing without rules of entry, you:

- identify the out-of-order factor,
- observe coincidental signals,
- find wisdom in the obstruction,

❖ discover past and future interconnectedness,

❖ become open to epiphanies, and

❖ commit to feedforward celebrations for what remains
to unfold in your future.

The most important insight you can gain, however, is to recognize there is *past* and *future* interconnectedness with your *present* experience of the drift. In other words, a synchronistic event encompasses past, present, and future meaningful coincidences, but we only look at how what happens in the present has coincidental meaning with the past, and we don't recognize that there is more to come in the future. To illustrate, in the example of the detoured flight, I only covered the past conditions leading to the present synchronicity; both people take the same flight to Rio (past) and fortuitously meet at the restaurant (present) where the synchronicity unfolds. But if they also celebrate a feedforward at the restaurant, they entangle the soon-to-unfold coincidences interconnected with their future! Hence, the out-of-order event is the entrance portal, and the feedforward celebration predisposes you to identify the future side of synchronicity.

The drift seems mysterious and difficult to grasp because of its simultaneous causes and their undetectable origins. You can readily determine the cause and *travel origin* of a linear path because it has detectable progression. For example, when you drive fifteen miles to work, the cause of your driving is to reach your place of employment, and home is the location where your trip originated. There is direct tracking from points A to B. But when you have simultaneous causes coming from multiple origins, you have what I call *indeterminate locality,* nonlinear pathways of multiple localities that are not accessible until they converge into linear perception. In other words, you can recognize the result, but not the cause and travel origin—analogous to a memory emerging apparently out of nowhere. But rather than "nowhere," the cause and travel origin have indeterminate locality. Although we feel like we weave in and out of the drift, we're always in it because interconnectedness is *intermittent* in our minds and *constant* in our world.

THE NAVIGATIONAL TOOLS

Although the drift is always with you, it is not something you can find at will. The tools I am going to teach you will help you recognize potential portals of entry, enter them, and navigate their synchronicity. The best way to proceed after you learn how to use the tools is to apply them without any expectations and go on about your life knowing there is interconnectedness in all you do. But there is no need to constantly be aware of the drift because you have other beautiful experiences and coauthors of love to enjoy on your journey. Rather than trying to *find* the drift, let it *invite* you to confirm you're not alone. Rather than a thing or entity, the drift is our collective human fabric that surfaces as islands of serenity in the middle of our storms.

<><><><><><><><><><><><><><><>

Setting the Stage

❖ Find a quiet place to relax and learn without distractions. Observe how your mindbody slows down.

❖ Recall a recent out-of-order event in your life and review how you handled the disruption. For example, one evening the electricity in your house suddenly went out. Did you avoid, resist, or enter the situation blindly? What would you do differently now?

❖ Reassess the out-of-order event and see if you detected, then or now, any meaningful coincidences. With no television to watch, as you usually do in the evenings, you grab a deck of cards, your spouse lights some candles, and you play a few hands of poker. If you're not mindful of the opportunities, synchronicities will go unnoticed.

❖ If you do not detect any synchronicity, allow yourself to speculate on what could have been one you missed, and if it does not surface immediately, allow it time to unfold, without forcing the issue. This speculation exercise helps you sharpen your detection skills. Don't be afraid to overinterpret the circumstances.

❖ Have a feedforward celebration relating to the out-of-order event. For example, go out to dinner to celebrate something fortuitous that will unfold that is interconnected with the out-of-order event. Do not speculate on *what* will unfold. Simply celebrate and let it go.

❖ Commit to viewing out-of-order events as opportunities to engage the drift. This does not mean you have to like what is happening. The wisdom you extract and the synchronicity you can engage have nothing to do with the emotional quality of the out-of-order event.

◇◇◇◇◇◇◇◇◇◇◇◇◇◇◇◇◇◇◇◇◇◇◇◇◇◇◇◇

Navigating the Drift

❖ Imagine an out-of-order condition. Use something stressful you may have to face in the near future. Approach it as if you're writing a story. For example, you suddenly learn you must immediately travel to someplace you have never been.

❖ When you choose the out-of-order condition, observe how your mindbody responds and take a couple of deep breaths from your belly without moving your shoulders. Observe the mindbody manifestations before moving on.

❖ Enter the out-of-order condition and begin to look for familiar aspects and potential guides. For example, if you are in a strange part of town, look for structures, colors, or anything else that reminds you of something familiar. Imagine a déjà vu. This familiarizing exercise tells your brain to send calming signals to your body. Potential guides could be friendly people or symbols that can direct your navigation.

❖ Repeat slowly like a mantra, "I have been here before," and recall memories of similar experiences in your life. What are the similarities and how did you handle the situation?

❖ Whatever you did before, imagine doing it more creatively. This exercise facilitates access to your experiential wisdom hidden in your memory archives, and improves it.

❖ Allow interconnectedness to enter your mindbody space. Observe what unfolds. Let the information come to you. Don't worry if you don't notice anything. It will come when you need it and learn to let go.

❖ Imagine that the drift, not your intellect, is guiding your intuition. Take steps based on what you sense, not on what you think or feel. Sensing has survival codes that have been refined for millennia.

❖ Recall times when your intuition guided you safely out of turbulence. How does the memory manifest in your mindbody? Observe and let go.

❖ Come out of the imagined situation and contemplate what you experienced. Recall the sequence of events and notice how it's expressed in your mindbody. Observe and let it pass.

❖ Commit to a feedforward celebration. Celebrate alone or with someone who can accept gracefully your "weird" celebration.

◇◇

Rituals to Invite Synchronicity

❖ At the end of each week, look for out-of-order conditions you did not notice. This exercise sharpens your mindfulness for the interconnectedness in your life.

❖ At least twice a month, have a feedforward celebration. Do not look for the future interconnectedness. It will come to you.

❖ Identify coauthors who obstruct or resist your celebrations. This does not mean people have to like or join you in your celebrations. It is rather to identify who is reluctant to share future joy with you.

❖ After the reason for your celebration unfolds in the future, allow yourself to feel gratitude for what you are learning about yourself and for accepting your right to be joyful.

❖ If you have someone *worthy* in your life who is reluctant to join you in your feedforward celebration, wait until the reason unfolds in the future and celebrate the known reason with that person. If that person refuses to celebrate the now-known reason,

look for other killjoy qualities this person may be
interjecting into your life.

❖ Be selective in sharing this information, but if you find
someone who is open to exploring, have a feedforward
celebration with that person and look for mutual
interconnectedness when either of you detects the
unfolding in the future. For example, if either of you
finds the individual reason for the celebration, see if it
also has a connection with the other person. This exercise
teaches you to expand your personal interconnected
mindfulness by including others.

<><><><><><><><><><><><><><><><><><><><><><><><><><><><><><><><><><><><><>

Engaging Negative Out-of-Order Events

❖ Recall a painful out-of-order event: something that
remains emotionally unresolved or seems random or
without reason.

❖ Experience the mindbody manifestation of the memory
and allow it to pass without interfering—like a moving
cloud on the horizon.

❖ Define the condition intellectually. For example, an
unexpected betrayal by a person you loved, someone
you trusted, and it deeply surprised you to realize this
person was not who you thought.

❖ Use the apophatic tool to negate anything you can
think about this person. For example, he/she is not bad,
not good, not trustworthy, not loving, not hating, not
friend, not enemy, not man, not woman, and so on,
until you run out of adjectives. Remember, apophatic

negation does not mean denial. It is a way of turning off the endless categorizing.

❖ Experience what you feel when you exhaust the negating labels. If new labels come up, repeat the apophatic process again until you exhaust your labels.

❖ Ask yourself, "If this person is not all the labels I could imagine, then who is this person?" Notice what you feel, and see if other labels come up. If they do, repeat the apophatic process again until you run out of labels.

❖ Once you reach a state void of categories, allow yourself to experience the void and notice what you feel. Allow the space void of labels to expand. Permit yourself to feel the serenity that comes when you disengage the need to categorize.

❖ Commit to a feedforward celebration.

◇◇◇◇◇◇◇◇◇◇◇◇◇◇◇◇◇◇◇◇◇◇◇◇◇◇◇◇◇◇◇◇◇

Extracting Creativity from Out-of-Order Events

❖ Recall an out-of-order event: something that remains emotionally unresolved or seems random or without reason.

❖ Experience the mindbody manifestation of the memory and allow it to pass without interfering, like a moving cloud on the horizon.

❖ Bring the unresolved or not-understood aspect of the experience to mind. Replay it until the circumstances are clear. Experience the mindbody response.

* Imagine you are ten years into the future and that you already know the resolution. Do not try to come up with a resolution or clarity. Just imagine you already know, and experience how that feels. This prolepsis tool allows you to access resolutions before their time in your history.

* Smile at the simplicity of the problem, now that you have solved it. Continue the experience without trying to find the solution. Imagine you are celebrating knowing the solution. It's analogous to knowing that you know without having to explain it—a precursor of knowledge. You are creating fertile ground for an unknown sprouting.

* Now allow your creativity to run wild and imagine solutions and answers to your questions without analyzing their feasibility or logic. Let credible and incredible answers flow without judging their merit.

* Notice what you feel as you're streaming solutions and answers. Avoid interpreting the practicality of the answers you imagine. For example, Einstein's dream about riding a rainbow helped him formulate his theory of relativity.

* Drop all the solutions and imagine you have a better one. Don't try to come up with a new solution; simply experience imagining that you know a better solution.

* See yourself fifteen years into the future and imagine how your life is. It does not have to be related to the answers you are seeking. The purpose is to let your mind travel to a place where logic does not allow it to go.

❖ Smile at how much you worried about something that now appears irrelevant because you solved the issue years ago. Continue to not look for answers. You're enjoying knowing without concern for what you know.

❖ See if you came up with novel answers or solutions. The point of the exercise is to open new registries of creativity. Whether now or later, you will find novel resolutions by practicing this exercise.

❖ Any time the memory of the unresolved out-of-order event comes up, take a deep breath from your stomach and imagine you already have the answer. Say to yourself, "I already know the answer," and let it go. You will either find a novel answer or be at peace knowing that you know the answer at a deeper level.

❖ Commit to a feedforward celebration and enjoy waiting, without expectations, for the unfolding of the celebrated knowing.

I suggest you practice often what you learned in this chapter to gain competence in navigating out-of-order events in your life. All the exercises are mindbody strategies to access creativity, wisdom, and novelty from your out-of-order experiences. The tools break from conventional access to memories and cognitive strategies to let your brain excel beyond the pale. Your cultural brain is learning a new subculture of excellence and hope.

❖ ❖ ❖

In the next chapter, I'll teach you how to create subcultures of wellness to support what you wish to incorporate from what you learned in this book. We are social beings and need confirmation and support from people we can respect and honor. We inherit our families and choose our friends, but this does not mean they will necessarily support our explorations of excellence beyond the pale. Don't blame them when they fail to support your journey of wellness, but don't let them stop you from reaching your worthy goals.

Creating Subcultures
of Wellness

You are by now fully aware that we are all coauthors of our triumphs as well as our miseries. Yet when we choose to grow emotionally, the path can be difficult—and for good reason. The people in our lives who have served as the coauthors of our dysfunctional patterns may not be ready for us to change. Instead, they may resort to emotional sabotage and other fear-based behaviors to maintain their collective but familiar misery.

A *subculture of wellness*, in contrast, opens opportunities to become your own best friend, share your excellence without fear of banishment, learn from mentors of wellness, and relinquish the legacy of unworthiness that has diminished the quality of your life.

To create sustainable change, you need cultural support. Applying the principles of cultural anthropology, I will teach you ways to break free of negative tribal patterns and create subcultures of wellness that support your emotional growth.

Please understand that creating subcultures of wellness does not necessarily mean you have to pack up and leave your home and family. What you have to *leave* is the self-entrapment patterns you were taught, independent of where you are and whom you are with.

SUBCULTURES BEYOND THE PALE

We are more than Darwinian survival-of-the-fittest beings. We are more predisposed to seek individual meaning than to propagate the species. We are more inclined to explore our personal excellence than live in mediocrity. And although we plan and build as if we are to live forever, we do so inspired by compassion rather than motivated by greed.

Then why is there so much suffering? Because, as I discussed in chapter 6, all cultures, with differing levels of intensity, invest in keeping their members nearsighted, teaching them to work for the collective needs of the tribe rather than find the hidden gifts that can transform an ordinary existence into one filled with an abundance of love, health, and wealth.

Fortunately, the boundaries of fear that tribes impose can be recontextualized into horizons of opportunity. If you have coauthored dysfunctional pathways with cultural editors who are invested in the false safety of known misery, you can also coauthor sustainable wellness within subcultures that love to celebrate your personal excellence.

By now you know I like to fly with poetics before landing on practicality. Aristophanes, a playwright of ancient Athens, said it best: "By words the mind is winged." I believe science does not have to be pedantically boring. But although words can take our minds to beautiful places, we have to embody our worthiness and coauthor our wellness if we wish to live there joyfully.

FROM BORDERS OF DEPRIVATION
TO HORIZONS OF ABUNDANCE

Subcultures of wellness are those that explore all the ways individual excellence can contribute to collective abundance. Your focus shifts away from remaining within the pale that keeps you trapped in collective known misery, and shifts toward freedom from the pale. Imagine a subculture that rejoices in your accomplishments and good fortune; envy is replaced with what Tibetan Buddhists call *empathic joy*. This is an expansive concept of joy and is a powerful antidote to envy. Empathic joy teaches you to relish the achievements of others as your own, and allows you to celebrate your good fortune without fear of banishment from the tribe. You no longer have to justify your unique accomplishments, personal excellence, and self-caring actions. Then, when you take yourself out to dinner for a personal celebration and the maître d' asks, "Only one?" you can exuberantly respond, "Yes!" without feeling the need to justify yourself.

I am not suggesting here that you should only celebrate by yourself. In subcultures of wellness, there are myriad ways to commemorate success.

Borders of Deprivation

Before we begin creating horizons of abundance, let's examine what it is that maintains the borders of deprivation. What is the fabric of these constraining limits?

One of the ways governments, institutions, and tribes maintain their power is by manipulating the concept of deprivation. The powers that be are invested in maintaining individual helplessness, and one way they do this is by ascribing nobility to poverty and malice to wealth. Personal excellence is viewed as arrogance; failure is attributed to external forces; and envy, resentment, and jealousy are rationalized as circumstances caused by the wealthy. What I am unfolding here is not a political stance. Instead, I am presenting the anthropological and sociological dynamics of power as studied extensively by Michel Foucault, Pierre Bourdieu, Maurice Merleau-Ponty, and other luminaries in the humanities and social sciences. Please stay with me while I explain each of the concepts I am proposing.

The Manipulation of Poverty

If you are poor, and you accept the premise that poverty is noble and wealth is evil, would you want to give up your nobility and become evil? In truth, socioeconomics has nothing whatever to do with character; individuals create morality or immorality independent of their economic conditions. Deprivation is best battled with earned access to resources, not with unearned handouts. To conclude that poverty is noble and wealth is evil absolves those who are poor and evil, and punishes those who are wealthy and noble. As is true, from rats to humans, *if you don't invest in what you wish to obtain, it loses value when you obtain it.*

Studies done with rats show that if they are given food without having to work for it, the food loses value for them. When they are given a choice to work for the food or not to, the rats consistently choose to earn their keep. It's the same for humans. Why? Because the effort you invest in a desired objective increases the value of the outcome. I will explain the value of *ownership* in the practical applications section at the end of the chapter.

The Punishment of Personal Excellence

If you were to work diligently, achieve your goals of excellence, and commit to leaving your world better than you found it, how would you feel if your achievements were seen as arrogant or selfish? Would you feel comfortable openly reveling in what you accomplished? What would happen if your cultural editors told you that if you failed, it must be because you relied on your own abilities rather than depending on your tribe? If you accepted the notion that the only way to win without being perceived as arrogant is to depend on your tribe, would you be willing to freely explore your individual abilities? Cultural editors who accept power from their tribes must coauthor conditions that facilitate individual excellence. But it is important to recognize that there are two types of power: one taken by force and one bestowed through admiration. Forced power is dictatorial and based in fear; bestowed power is benevolent and based in love. You may recall from chapter 3 that the two powers have different psychoneuroimmunological effects. Force dictates helplessness, while admiration facilitates empowerment.

The Manipulation of Envy, Resentment, and Jealousy

The powerful who perpetuate dependence find great value in manipulating the fear-based emotions that lead to unworthiness. Envy, resentment, and jealousy are fed by deprivation and imposed collectivism. Why? Because, if you believe your achievements are flawed when they occur beyond the pale, you need the emotions of envy, resentment, and jealousy to rationalize coveting what others achieved when they took risks beyond the pale—while you remained safely within walls. These fear-based emotions are very effective in keeping you from exploring your excellence.

When others achieve beyond our set limits of abundance, we are left with two choices: to rationalize our unworthiness with fear-based emotions that we project onto the achiever, or to find the courage to emulate the achiever. There is a third choice if you don't want to succumb to envy or invest in whatever may be required to obtain what others have: you can appreciate the achiever's accomplishment as if it were your own. In the practical applications section of this chapter, I will show you how to apply empathic joy and other antidotes to resolve your fear-based emotions.

Horizons of Abundance

I hope you are continuing to discover that although many biocognitive principles are counterintuitive, they are powerful agents of change. It's also important to recognize that most of the cultural controls I address in this chapter are strategies that originally had tribal value for collective conservation and well-being, and were not necessarily based on malicious intent. Instead, these controls lost their initial value because they did not expand to accommodate positive contextual changes.

When the automobile was commercialized, there were massive protests, even riots, led by coachmen who feared the introduction of the taxicab as a technological evil that would put an end to their trade. Some politicians, in order to manipulate this collective fear, vilified the automobile in support of coachmen and the builders of horse-driven carriages. Coachmen who did not succumb to the political manipulation of their "helplessness" learned to drive taxis, and progressive companies that built horse-driven carriages saw the opportunity to manufacture automobiles.

When you first encounter the horizons of abundance, they may strike you as obstructions because they require a shift in operative consciousness before you can see their potential benefits. You might see boundaries of deprivation rather than opportunities, but when you're faced with the end of "business as usual," you can choose to recontextualize it as an opportunity to explore your next level of abundance. You can thrive where others get stuck.

FINDING MENTORS IN SUBCULTURES OF WELLNESS

Creating subcultures of wellness is essential if you are to transcend the tribal boundaries your cultural editors taught you to respect. Anthropological research shows that tribes that support wellness have cultural editors who gained their power through admiration, not by imposing fear. One of your tasks is to replace the cultural editors who taught you unworthiness with mentors you can admire and wish to emulate.

Cultural editors shape your self-valuation early in life, when you must depend on them for physical, emotional, and intellectual nourishment. You learned in chapter 2 that most people are willing to pay the price of archetypal wounds in order to get the love they need. The new subculture of wellness that you will create requires a different language of love. You needed the cultural editors of the old tribe yet lacked the ability to choose the good and reject the bad. In subcultures of wellness, *you* choose your mentors rather than letting them choose you. When you create subcultures of wellness, you untangle love from your archetypal wounds and select mentors based on your own worthiness rather than on the unworthiness you were taught "for your own good."

RELINQUISHING THE COMFORT OF COMPLIANCE

Replacing the comfort of known misery with the discomfort of unknown joy can be one of the main obstacles on your path to wellness. Although you may want the joy of personal freedom, learned dependence has its hidden advantages. It diminishes your risks and lets you disown responsibility, instead relying on others to make your tough decisions for you.

Most Western mythologies have stories of heroes and Titans who paid a dear price for defying the gods or their cultural editors. According to Greek mythology, Prometheus revealed to humanity the secret of creating fire, and then was eternally condemned by the gods to endure the daily agony of an eagle devouring his liver. At the end of each day, Prometheus grew a new liver, perpetuating his punishment. Sisyphus, another Greek hero, revealed the secret of immortality to mankind and was compelled to roll an immense boulder up a hill, only to watch it roll back down—and repeat the task forever. Icarus was given wings of wax by his father, but when the young man flew too close to the god of the sun, the wings melted, and he fell to his death. Although Native American, Eastern, and African myths depict deities with more tolerance for their heroes, most cultures have admonitions to prevent their members from excelling beyond what the tribe considers prudent.

We have long tribal histories that relentlessly set limits on what we can achieve without offending the collective wisdom. And although we don't have to deal with mythical deities, we are still vulnerable to tribal archetypal wounding to dissuade us from venturing beyond the pale. I have belabored the power of tribes in order to help you identify the many masks they wear. The French philosopher Michel Foucault dedicated his professional life to studying the origin and dynamics of power. He warned that societal controls are so deeply embedded in our consciousness that we function as if we were in a fish tank, unable to see the glass that contains us.

TAKING THE WISDOM OF YOUR TRIBE TO YOUR SUBCULTURE OF WELLNESS

Not everything about tribes is bad. They evolved as a result of millennia of human misery and devastating, turbulent conditions. The task is to find the wisdom underlying the survival of your tribe while discarding what is no longer functional for you.

Let's start with the wisdom of bonding to make a group stronger than any of its individuals. Bonding can be functional or dysfunctional based on contextual circumstances. Reasons for healthy bonding include guarding against evil, protecting the weak, and recognizing individual excellence. Reasons for unhealthy bonding include permitting abuse of the innocent, promoting fear, and punishing individual excellence. Foucault's metaphor of the fish tank can help you see through the glass that encloses your culture. But to avoid taking dysfunctional patterns from the tribe into your subculture of wellness, you must recognize that the power that forcibly controlled you indirectly taught you how to control yourself and others forcibly. In your subculture of wellness, you can substitute healthy bonding, bestowed power, and horizons of abundance for the glass enclosures of deprivation. However, before you can coauthor your subculture of wellness, you must relinquish the forced-power methods you learned from your dysfunctional editors.

COAUTHORING YOUR SUBCULTURE OF WELLNESS

Now that you understand what has kept you in your tribal fish tank, you can create greater freedom and a better life using your newfound wisdom. Be sure to carefully coauthor your subculture of wellness to avoid bringing with you unhelpful patterns and unwanted teachers. If you are not mindful of your history when you enter a new environment, it's all too easy to slip back into known misery.

Let's look at what you need to avoid when you want to coauthor wellness. Along with Foucault's fish tank to remind you of the invisible constraints of your tribe, unmasking the enemies of wellness is another metaphor you can use on your new journey. Cultural editors disguise their forcible control as benevolence to make the constraints they impose on you appear as if they were intended for your own good. Let's begin the unmasking.

◇◇◇◇◇◇◇◇◇◇◇◇◇◇◇◇◇◇◇◇◇◇◇◇◇◇◇◇◇◇◇◇◇◇◇◇

The Within-the-Pale Mask

If it were up to your cultural editors, you would never leave the tribe. The pale that constrains you is invisible and strong, like armored glass; you cannot break through if you are not aware of how you have inadvertently assimilated your enclosure. Realizing that the enclosure is a *learned option* can help you unlearn it. Before you attempt to leave the pale, recognize that its initial function was to protect you as a member of the tribe. Cultural editors can be as unaware of the controls they impose on you as you are unaware of the constraining effects their power has on your life. Tribes are classrooms of blinded teachers delivering blind lessons: a coauthoring of inadvertent knowing.

Never leave the tribe with resentment. Instead, celebrate the fact that you have the option to leave. And remember that it's not always necessary to leave a person or place physically. Yes, you can leave a person or place if your worthiness is not supported there, but you can also leave an old pattern of unworthiness and remain where you are, as long as your new pattern of worthiness is supported. Subcultures of wellness are conditions of support you coauthor with people who are willing to accept your worthiness. In other words, leaving the tribe can be physical or conceptual.

❖ Identify your fear of leaving your tribe and where your apprehension manifests in your body. Do you feel tightness in your chest or shallow breathing? Breathe deeply and observe without judging the manifestations. You are simply experiencing the response your mindbody learned when you presented it with options to expand your horizons. When you are confronted with unknown contexts, the turbulence you experience is normal. The brain is trying to decide whether to accept or reject a new condition. The turbulence subsides when you decide what to do.

❖ The tribal pale is symbolic. Although you feel enclosed, there are no physical boundaries. Imagine an area you want to explore: new friends, different work, new relationships. As you consider these new conditions, see if someone comes to mind who may want to stop you or who may demand explanations for what you are trying to change.

❖ After unmasking your self-imposed constraints and the coauthors who perpetuate your limitations within the pale, celebrate what you have learned and take your first steps beyond the pale.

The Deprivation Mask

There is no joy in forced deprivation. It teaches learned helplessness, which is bad for your health. Glorifying and honoring deprivation create a false sense of comfort to keep you in known misery. You unmask deprivation when you coauthor conditions that are incompatible with unworthiness.

* Look for patterns you are using to limit your own joy, such as procrastination, unrealistic goals, blaming others, and so on. When you unmask the culprit, pay attention to how your body responds. Breathe gently and observe your mindbody reactions. Celebrate with simple rituals what you have learned: go for a walk, break bread with a coauthor of wellness, meditate, show gratitude, or discover something new in your old habits. Once you make the commitment to celebrate, don't break it. Celebrate as soon as possible; waiting for more than a few days allows your old dysfunctional patterns to weaken your good intentions, and the probability of self-sabotage increases significantly.

* Look for ways in which others limit your joy, and when you can see their toxic strategies, set protective limits. If they do not respect the limits you set, do not invite the violators to your subculture of wellness. Assertiveness has two steps: setting limits *and* giving permission for others to not like your limits. If you exclude the second step of assertiveness, you will revert to your previous limits because you chose to be liked rather than respected.

I used joy as the working theme in this exercise to introduce you to another biocognitive tool: *indirect incompatibility*. You can replace your dysfunctional patterns with conditions that are directly or indirectly incompatible with what you are trying to change. Joy is *indirectly* incompatible with deprivation because joy is an expression of abundance. And since abundance is the opposite of deprivation, joy is indirectly incompatible with deprivation.

Why should you use indirect tools to change dysfunctional patterns? Because under certain conditions, direct tools are not immediately accessible or simple to apply. In the example of using joy rather than abundance to change patterns of deprivation, it's easier to access joy than to create the abundance you want. To make this new tool easier to understand, I will use it again later to unmask other enemies of wellness.

◇◇◇◇◇◇◇◇◇◇◇◇◇◇◇◇◇◇◇◇◇◇◇◇◇◇

The Bonding Mask

The initial functions of bonding with a group are to protect you and establish your tribal identity. The mask comes into use when the initial noble intentions of bonding are disguised to impose forced power. The bonding mask presents forced constraints, as if they were benevolent attempts to protect you from external dangers. What began as an authentic attempt to protect you becomes the protection of collective power at your expense. Let's begin to unmask dysfunctional bonding.

❖ Look for coauthors who protected you when you were a child but lost their function when you no longer needed protection as an adult. For example, a parent who continues to tell you how to live your life. Imagine circumstances in which you could be your own protector. Who will lose their jobs as your protectors if you protect yourself? How do you unwittingly facilitate the role of protectors you no longer need? How does your body respond when you imagine these scenarios? Breathe and observe how you are unmasking dysfunctional bonds.

❖ After you rehearse unmasking dysfunctional bonds using imagery, take *ownership* of your self-protection role when you enact it in the subculture of wellness you are creating. You take ownership of protection when you *feel* the mindbody meaning of investing in your own protection. For example, when you experience what you feel the moment you take action to protect yourself, you *own* that action. Conversely, when someone else protects you, you feel that you are being protected—you have no ownership of what takes place. As I mentioned earlier, ownership brings value to your mindbody investments. Valuing your actions is another way to create indirect incompatibility with your unworthy patterns. As you apply these concepts you will notice, with increasing frequency, the interrelatedness of biocognitive principles.

◇◇◇◇◇◇◇◇◇◇◇◇◇◇◇◇◇◇◇◇◇◇◇◇◇◇◇◇◇◇◇◇◇◇◇◇◇◇◇

INSIDE YOUR SUBCULTURE OF WELLNESS

You now know how to break out of your tribal fish tank and enter a subculture of wellness. Within your subculture, you will live alongside coauthors keen on celebrating individual excellence, as well as mentors who earn their bestowed power, bonding without hidden agendas, and owning personal worthiness without fear of banishment. But keep in mind that you are not trying to create paradise. Life is more exciting than perfect! Navigate your journey with the courage and resilience to avoid chasing winds of hope that cannot be harnessed. Perfection is an illusion, self-defined enlightenment is mystical narcissism, and running away to a cave while there's hunger and suffering in the world is spiritual selfishness. It is best to seek imperfect teachers who earn your admiration for the elegance of their humility. So, rather than a panacea, in the next chapter I offer a compass for your private journey of self, to help you navigate your ocean without having to know every wave ahead of time. Celebrate the wisdom of your imperfections, and we'll meet again when you're ready to read on.

A Compass for the Private Journey of Self

In this concluding chapter, I will offer additional insights, building upon those you have already discovered in this book. I'll also introduce you to the internal compasses—as opposed to external maps imposed from without—you can use to navigate turbulence in all areas of your life. Learning to cope with problems in this way is important. Ultimately, however, in sharing the principles of biocognition, I aim to delineate a way of life that will empower you to successfully break through any barriers to wellness, clearing your path to an abundance of love, health, and wealth.

As we begin our discussion of internal compasses, let me underscore a theme you have seen repeatedly in this book. Your best intentions to change what does not serve you well are necessary, but intentions alone are not sufficient for you to achieve your worthy goals. Change is difficult to implement. This is because it will be challenged every step of the way by your own fears and by the cultural editors who have coauthored your present life and who will not stop trying to shape you in their own image simply because you have decided to change. As you encounter these obstacles to change, remember that the motives for what you did to yourself in the past, or allowed others to do to you, will cease to be important when you realize that, although your past has shaped you, the present moment always offers an invitation to heal.

THE USUAL SUSPECTS

Let's examine what your inner voice may say to you, and how others might respond, when you try to change. Imagine a dialogue with a friend.

> YOU "I recently read this book that gave me some new ideas, and some really unique tools to change things about my life that have bothered me for a long time. It's really an intriguing new system, and I'd like to try it. But using the tools takes practice, and I don't think I have enough time to do that."
>
> FRIEND "Yeah? Well, I've read a lot of self-help books myself, and I think they all say the same thing."
>
> YOU "Well this book is different from others I've read. For one thing, it tells you that being positive and having good intentions are not enough."
>
> FRIEND "So what else does it say you need?"
>
> YOU "The author teaches that you need to cultivate a sense of self-worth before you can truly accept the changes you're looking for."
>
> FRIEND "I don't know about that. I have great self-worth, and I still can't get out of my terrible marriage."
>
> YOU "Yeah, well, maybe this won't work either, but I think I'm going to give it a try and see what happens."
>
> FRIEND "Well, it's your time. Let me know how it goes."
>
> YOUR INNER DIALOGUE "Maybe she's right. I've also read a lot of books that said I'd get good results, and they didn't seem to help me. And I am really busy now . . . Maybe I'll give it a try when I have more time."

Failure Archetypes

In a dialogue like the preceding one, you and your friend are engaging in what I call *failure archetypes:* procrastination, cynicism, pessimism, and a sense of unworthiness. You can find all these in this conversation, but the following underlying dynamic may not be as obvious. When we share information about something new with one another, we tend to implicitly set it up so others can confirm our doubts. Here, this took the form of you telling your friend you learned something new, but you're not sure if you have time to practice it. In this way, you invited your friend to engage failure archetypes.

Interestingly, most of us are more willing to accept an invitation to maintain a status quo of failure than to forge into new territory and shake up our world with joy.

Success Archetypes

Just as the three archetypal wounds that you are now well acquainted with (abandonment, shame, and betrayal) have healing fields (commitment, honor, and loyalty), failure archetypes also have their counterparts. Failure archetypes are based on fear, and *success archetypes* are fed by love. Fear keeps you within the realm of your known misery; since the known is predictable, it provides pseudocomfort—misery with no surprises. Love propels you into the unknown joy that awaits you.

This is why I insist that we build our sense of self-worth *before* we explore abundance, which we can think of as *joy with surprises.* Fear threatens, while love entices, and we prioritize responding to menace before responding to persuasion. But what if you taught your cultural brain to view both fear and love as *invitations?* This is what they are. Both the danger of fear and the enticement of love are offers you may consider—and you may either accept or reject them.

If fear enslaves you in archetypes of procrastination, cynicism, pessimism, and unworthiness, love liberates you to live archetypes of commitment, trust, faith, and worthiness. Remember, both are *invitations* to navigate your private journey.

INTERNAL GUIDES FOR NAVIGATING TURBULENCE

Although you can recontextualize fear and love as invitations, you still need the benefit of a tool to move beyond wishful thinking and positive thinking. Staying with the metaphor of a journey, it's more important to know how to respond to something new than to know where you happened to find it; if you use a city map to find a street, it won't include instructions for what to do if you get mugged or seduced once you get there. So in this chapter, I'll teach you how to proceed under good and bad conditions alike, using a compass that responds to context instead of whereabouts.

Directional space has four cardinal points: north, south, east, and west. The private journey of self has three cardinal points—*patience, courage,* and *faith*—and to navigate, you need a compass that points to these three internal guides. As you know, all biocognitive tools are evidence-based, and the internal compass is no exception. Next I'll teach you when to access each of these three guides and present you with the evidence that validates them.

Choosing the Internal Guides

Your internal compass that points to patience, courage, and faith can guide you through any turbulence you encounter in your life, whether good or bad. Let me illustrate with some examples.

Let's say you fall in love with a wonderful person who has two young children from a previous relationship. You've already experienced being a parent and have never considered raising more children, yet this person has all the qualities you admire and have wished to find in a partner. This is *good* turbulence . . . that is beginning to look troublesome. Which of the three guides do you think you need?

To discover the appropriate guide for you in this situation, first identify your concerns. What surfaces when you consider the decision to commit again? (a) Are you intolerant of young children? (b) Are you unsure you can truly love again? (c) Do you fear failure in this relationship?

Although the three internal guides are interrelated, if you dig deeply enough you will *always* find that one fits best for each circumstance you face. In this example, for (a) you need to access the *patience* to share your life with children, for (b) the *faith* that new love is possible for you, and for (c) the *courage* to move toward joy despite your fear. There is no external map to lead you to the right choice; you will determine which compass point to follow subjectively, because the decision is colored by your cultural history.

For another case in point, say that your routine medical checkup shows you have high cholesterol and high blood pressure, and when you step on the scale you are startled to learn that you are twenty pounds overweight—again. Before considering any medication, your holistic doctor gives you a three-month protocol that includes substantial lifestyle changes. Then you talk to your mom, who reminds you there's a history of stroke on her side of the family. You've tried to lose weight and eat healthy diets before, but always gave up after a few weeks. Still, you really don't want to have to be on medication for the rest of your life.

You'll have to access patience in order to follow your doctor's advice. You'll need faith to try a new strategy that can improve your wellness. And you will need courage to defy your mom's message of being genetically sentenced to suffer a stroke. Of course, as a good biocognitive student, you know that intentions are not enough to achieve sustainable change. Evidence is the missing ingredient, and where do you find it?

You have already learned that forgiving and healing archetypal wounds have little to do with those who inflicted them upon you. It is the interpretation you make of the event that disempowers you, not the event itself. And since you make interpretations in your biocognitive space, that is where you resolve them. You look for any evidence of empowering experiences in the past (not necessarily related to the event), and when you embody the memory of those experiences, you recontextualize helplessness and thus regain self-worth. And as you may recall, recontextualizing changes the felt meaning of symbols, beliefs, and words.

This same process applies to finding evidence of patience, courage, and faith. For example, if you have determined that patience is what you need, you can recall instances when it served you well during turbulent times. Then, just as you have done throughout the exercises in this book, you embody what you feel when you replay the memory of choosing patience instead of haste. *This is evidence you already own.* Patience, courage, and faith empower you in the face of turbulence, while their counterparts—haste, timidity, and doubt—render you helpless. By recalling instances when your three inner guides worked well for you in other circumstances when you were faced with their counterparts, you can move from intention to action with more confidence that you will master your challenges.

If you are looking for evidence of the wisdom of patience, it can be as simple as recalling a time when you wanted to respond hastily to an email that angered you, but waited until your response could be more cogent and graceful; you chose the high road. All three inner guides give your brain enough time to transfer information from the primitive fight-or-flight area (the amygdala) to the socialized one (the left frontal lobe), where you can then make a wise decision you will not regret later. By the way, giving the guides time to work does not make you a pushover. Interestingly, using the inner compass will teach you to discern when it's appropriate to express righteous anger—which is one of the causes of health—to set limits.

DELINEATING THE MINDBODY CAUSES OF HEALTH

Now that you have a good foundation in biocognition, I can return to the most revolutionary concepts of this theory. I argue that:

❖ most illnesses are *learned,* and
❖ the causes of health are *inherited.*

There's overwhelming evidence that smokers *teach* their lungs susceptibility to cancer and emphysema. But what is not so obvious is that most other illnesses are learned as well. What I mean by "teach" here needs clarification. The lungs know what to do to keep their inner lining free of impurities. They produce mucus to engulf foreign bodies, and they clean them out with their broomlike cilia. But since smoking repeatedly fills the lungs with hot air that contains nicotine and many other toxic chemicals, the action "teaches" the lungs to overproduce mucus and slow down the cleaning mechanism. The toxic lesson continues and eventually results in illness. The lungs have been taught to get sick. This does *not* mean, however, that we *cause* our illnesses. Instead, in addition to the influence of environmental conditions and diets, our genetic predispositions become activated by the operative consciousness we present to our immune system, creating dysfunctional patterns that teach our mindbody how to break down.

What does this mean? In chapter 3, I proposed that the immune system is more than a network of protection because it also confirms the cultural beliefs we embody. If you live a life of generalized fear, your immune system reflects your helplessness and allows free rein to opportunistic pathogens. But you must *never* blame yourself if you have an illness. What I am suggesting here is very complex, and the process is not as straightforward as it appears. It is far more important to recognize that you've inherited a couple of million years of experience in refining the causes of your health. Why is this not obvious after all this time? Because most health sciences continue to focus on what makes us sick, not on all the ways we learn to be ill.

The model of pathology concludes that what makes us sick needs to be treated externally. Once pathology reaches a critical mass, reductionist medicine has no alternative but to intervene aggressively; there is no time for less intrusive options. And since it's so focused on detecting pathology, it neglects to explore the causes of mindbody health. I argue that, if you allow the internal causes of health to intervene early in the learning of an illness, you can prevent reaching a level of pathology that requires aggressive external intervention.

By the way, many health care professionals agree with what I am proposing but lack viable alternatives to intervene when pathology hits the fan. And it is imperative that I don't leave you with the impression that I am dismissing medical treatment; it would be naive and irresponsible for me to take such a radical stance.

It's not easy to criticize a science that saves lives. Having worked as a clinical neuropsychologist in mental health centers and hospitals, I can attest that many of the medical technologies and interventions I've witnessed are no less than stellar. Moreover, the dedication and knowledge of most health care professionals are beyond reproach. So, rather than replace the conventional health care model, I offer a perspective that can enhance it. I believe we should investigate what causes our health with the same fervor we bring to what makes us sick. The absence of one does not explain the other.

For instance, a virus *appears* to cause the common cold, but this interpretation confuses cause and effect because it assumes the virus is acting alone. The true cause is a *coauthoring* of the virus with a weak immune system. If you treat the viral infection, you help the immune system fight the virus, but the healing does not end there; the operational consciousness that keeps the immune system weak also needs to be addressed. If you neglect the conditions that permit the coauthoring of an illness, you can cure it only temporarily. You cannot achieve permanent healing.

You inherited the causes of health because millennia of mindbody refinements that enhance the effectiveness and efficiency of your immune system were passed on from one generation to the next. But it's important to understand that the immune system's cells and molecules have not changed much in the last several thousands of years. It is the refinement of our cognitions and emotions that allows the immune system to perform at its best. The immune system is the player, and our operative consciousness is the play. You have met these refinements earlier in this book: elevated cognitions and exalted emotions. The elevated cognitions include honor, commitment, loyalty, dignity, modesty, admiration, honesty, fairness, and magnanimity. And the exalted emotions include compassion, empathy, kindness, generosity, and gratitude.

These elevated cognitions and exalted emotions *are* the causes of health. They provide the *bonding* and *limit setting* necessary for our immune system to shine during our most challenging times.

Let me underscore this point, as it is novel and bears repeating: *our elevated cognitions and exalted emotions are the causes of our health.*

Although these emotions and cognitions each have their unique characteristics, they function in mindbody unison. For instance, the *cognition* of honor is inseparable from the embodied sensations and emotions it generates. Likewise, the *emotion* of compassion has sensations and cognitions that go along with it. These mindbody expressions are the product of our human refinement, and when they are experienced in their appropriate contexts, they create an ideal operative consciousness that the immune system can *confirm*—optimal conditions for mindbody wellness. I say "confirm" because, although your immune system is designed to protect you, it responds within the restrictions you impose when you confront life challenges. It's analogous to freeing or cuffing the hands that are trying to protect you. And although it seems like the immune system "conforms" to the limitations you impose, it's actually confirming the operative consciousness that you're teaching it.

What is the difference and why is it important? Because conforming means acquiescing to pressure, whereas confirming means validating or giving support. And I believe the immune system gives great relevance to your operative consciousness—even when it's not in your best interest. Initially, it continues to fight for you, but because it's a coauthoring student, it concludes that the dysfunctional lessons you're teaching it are the best way to go.

I need to point out that I am proposing a theoretical model of the immune system that is certainly open to scientific debate, but I believe this concept of confirmation can explain why the immune system breaks its own rules and begins to attack the self (manifesting as autoimmune disorders), overreact (allergy disorders), and underreact (immune deficiency disorders) when it should be protecting you. But once again, I caution you *not* to conclude this means you are causing your illnesses; this is very far from the truth. Instead, I propose that the good and bad lessons you teach your immune system interact with environmental conditions, diet, and genetic predispositions to collectively determine your health and illnesses.

FUNCTIONS OF THE MINDBODY CAUSES OF HEALTH

If we are to heal and stay healthy, we need to socially connect and set emotional limits, but in our socialization process we must apply the mindbody causes of health to ourselves as much as we do to others. This means each of the causes of health has to be inclusive. When you express compassion for others, you must include yourself in the process, and when you honor someone, you must also honor yourself. This inclusivity is what indirectly supports self-worth, self-caring, and self-protection.

For instance, Tibetan Buddhist psychology teaches that not including yourself in an act of compassion negates the legitimacy of that emotion. The best way to understand the kind of inclusiveness I refer to is to think about why, on an airplane, if there is a loss of cabin pressure, flight attendants instruct you to breathe first from your own oxygen mask before giving one to a child (a great lesson for caretakers).

In addition to their socialization value, the mindbody causes of health trigger biological responses that enhance immune function. In chapter 3, I discussed the health benefits of these responses and their reciprocal effect. Externally, they express behaviors that bring out the best in you to share with others. And internally, they create biochemistry that maximizes physical and emotional wellness. This powerful combination of mindbody wellness is available to you when you coauthor inclusive love.

Bonding

Our need to connect with, learn to get along with, and empathize with others is necessary to our survival. One of the best ways to conceptualize the importance of bonding is to recall a time when you disconnected from a loving relationship and your wellness diminished. You lost the reciprocal benefit of your loving relationship because loving and being loved are inseparable.

Where bonding is concerned, it's important to recognize the difference between isolating yourself for fear of loving others and protecting yourself from those whose love is entangled with archetypal wounds. How can you tell the difference? Fear leads to your withholding your love, whereas protective self-care rescues you from loving in the wrong places. It's healthier to suspend your love than to accept it from those who entangle it with shame, abandonment, and betrayal. However, if you're indifferent to the suffering and joy of those you choose to love, self-caring turns into self-centeredness, and healthy caretaking into selfishness. When you discontinue your empathic connections to others, you not only break bonds; you become an island of isolation, and you nullify your causes of health. Empathy and compassion are the qualities most conducive to reading what others feel.

Setting Emotional Limits

The inclusivity component of the mindbody causes of health helps us detect when our emotional limits are off balance; we feel guilty when we don't give enough, and resentful when we give too much. You can calibrate your emotional limits by using these two emotions. Just be aware that if you mostly function from either end of the scale, from guilt at one end to resentment at the other, there's a tendency to miscalculate the *opposite* side of the scale.

For example, when you're used to living with guilt, it's difficult to express resentment. This is why victims have difficulty calibrating the resentment side, and martyrs have problems with the guilt side. Interestingly, too much caretaking leads to a disorder called *empathic fatigue*. It has the same symptoms as burnout but a different cause. Without self-caring limits, the workaholic archetype leads to burnout, and the caretaking type leads to empathic fatigue. If the overused archetype is not contextually balanced, a simple solution like taking a vacation will only relieve symptoms. When archetypes are chronically experienced beyond their function, they promote illness. Living from a single archetype, regardless of context, is analogous to using a hammer no matter what needs fixing, even to tighten a screw.

Benign Boundaries

Like all the mindbody processes I introduce in this book, the causes of health function harmoniously when we express them from the middle way: the Buddhist psychology concept meaning the optimal position between opposites—not bitter/not sweet, not hot/not cold, and so on. Once you determine your boundaries, you have to give others permission to not like them. It's important to recognize that you coauthored whatever you are now trying to limit, and just because you're ready to make changes does not mean you will get the support you expect. When you're feeling abused because your boundaries are not respected, you may need righteous anger to feel worthy of your self-caring stance. This type of anger is contextual, never to be used outside of circumstances when you feel abused.

By definition, righteous anger is righteous because it arises when you're protecting your innocence, generosity, or goodwill. It's the only kind of anger that enhances immune function and general wellness. But remember, if it's taken out of context, it turns into a toxic anger that can make you sick. Inclusivity and righteous anger are the ingredients for balancing your mindbody causes of health.

HOW TO ACCESS THE MINDBODY
CAUSES OF HEALTH

As we have seen, the context of your situation determines which causes of health you need to access in order to heal disharmony and maintain wellness. I introduce the concept of disharmony here to illustrate how the causes of health can recontextualize learned illnesses.

An illness is a dysfunctional learning process that results in a critical pathological mass—a disruption of systemic harmony. Conventional medicine identifies the "measurable" pathology of illness but fails to see that the cause is the end product of *learned disharmony*. This dysfunctional learning remains underground, where chronic helplessness takes root; it is from these roots that pathology sprouts. But knowing that illness is learned more than acquired will allow you to intervene before it's too late.

You can also access your causes of health after illness surfaces by unlearning the disharmony. Before I explain how to intervene in this way, I want you to know that I am well aware that when some illnesses reach a critical mass, neither medical intervention nor the causes of health, nor both together, are sufficient to reverse the damage. Nevertheless, there is much you can do if you are ill, without losing hope or blaming yourself.

The way to access the causes of health is the same for healing as it is for maintaining wellness. Unfortunately, we are more willing to implement needed change when illness strikes than when we are healthy, so I want to encourage you to break that pattern. Then you will be able to catch any lurking dysfunctional learning before it expresses itself in mindbody pathology.

The Assessments Tools

Before you can determine the appropriate causes of health, you have to identify the area(s) of disharmony in your life—the patterns of imbalance.

Areas of Disharmony

There are two main area of disharmony to consider:

Bonding—The degree and quality of connections with family, friends, and work environments.

Limits—The degree of benign boundaries set with family members, friends, and coworkers.

Are you experiencing difficulty in connecting with others, setting limits, or both? How long have you been experiencing disharmony in this area? Who are the coauthors you need to embrace or confront? What do you fear about taking corrective action? These same questions serve as the assessment tools you need whether you are trying to maintain or restore wellness. If you are recovering from an illness, they help you identify what to incorporate in your existing treatment plan, and if you are healthy, what to correct before disharmonious learning reaches a pathological critical mass.

Again, I cannot emphasize enough that these interventions enhance, rather than replace, the treatment prescribed by your health care professionals.

The Tools for Restoring Harmony

After you identify the area(s) of disharmony, you will choose the mindbody causes of health that are best suited to restore balance. You will also determine which internal guide(s) you need to confront the turbulence of change. Let's look at a few examples to help you navigate the balancing process. You can scan the outline that follows to help you determine which tools to use.

Compass Points: Your Internal Guides

Courage—This is the compass point to follow to overcome conditions in which fear is affecting your social, professional, emotional, physical, and spiritual wellness.

Patience—Aim for this heading if haste, toxic anger, and arrogance surface when you confront a challenge.

Faith—This is your guide when cynicism, pessimism, negativity, and prior failures are keeping you from reaching worthy goals.

The Causes of Health

Elevated Cognitions—The honor, commitment, loyalty, dignity, modesty, admiration, honesty, fairness, and magnanimity required to gracefully confront your challenges.

Exalted Emotions—The compassion, empathy, kindness, generosity, and gratitude required to lovingly confront your challenges.

Balancing Tools for the Causes of Health

Inclusivity—Including yourself in the elevated cognitions and exalted emotions you express to others.

Righteous Anger—Appropriate indignation when others abuse your innocence, generosity, or goodwill. Righteous anger is also justified when others abuse those you love.

❖ ❖ ❖

Now let's look at how you might use these tools in practice. Let's suppose that you've determined that *bonding* is off balance in your life. You've gradually isolated yourself from people you love because you fear getting hurt again. Since *fear* is the blocking agent, *courage* is the internal guide you need, and *empathy* is the exalted emotion for the cause of health. *Inclusivity* is the tool you bring to bear to extend this exalted emotion to yourself.

If you are in the phase of restoring your health, you can also determine whether your fear was caused by an archetypal wound. If it was, you can include the elevated cognition that resolves it (honor for shame, commitment for abandonment, and loyalty for betrayal).

You can see how different areas come together to enhance the causes of health and consequently your immune system. You integrate internal guides (compass points), the mindbody causes of health, and archetypal healing fields. These are powerful allies of wellness.

As another example, you find that *limit setting* is your area of disharmony. You recognize that a loved one is abusing your generosity, and you're resenting the intrusion. You also realize you have been caretaking this person and neglecting your own emotional needs. Since you understand the concept of coauthoring, you don't waste time blaming the other person. Instead, you move forward armed with the limit-setting tools of inclusivity and, if needed, righteous anger. In this situation, your generosity is being abused, and you're not respecting your need to take time for yourself. It becomes clear to you that when you allow others to disrespect your limits, your coauthoring includes not respecting your own. You decide the balancing act requires the inner guide of courage to confront your abuser, righteous anger to propel your corrective action, and the elevated cognition of fairness to prevent you from responding in a self-destructive way as a distraction—for example, by overeating.

I hope you can see the wealth of permutations you can create to correct every kind of disharmony in your life!

BEYOND THE LESSONS

Biocognitive tools are designed to work synergistically with one another so that the sum is always greater than the parts. Correcting one area of disharmony has unexpected benefits that may not be obvious when you're choosing the path to take. For example, in the process of restoring bonding balance, you may need to establish benign limits and heal archetypal wounds. These tools enter the pathways of your mindbody complex to enhance healing and prevent further damage from the underlying dysfunctional learning patterns that can lead to illness.

The causes of health have always been within you. They're your birthright, available to you the moment you take time to assess what you need in order to achieve sustainable wellness while remaining a guardian of the heart to those you choose to love. Coauthoring embraces balance, and self-love is the balancing act.

❖ ❖ ❖

As you turn the last pages of this book, I invite you to take stock of the knowledge you have gained. You now know how tribes teach through their designated cultural editors, how to untangle love from archetypal wounds, how longevity is learned, how relationships heal, and how to excel beyond the pale without having to pay the tribal price. You know that all these patterns of healthy change require you to join subcultures of wellness that confirm the best in you and that coauthor environments that are simply incompatible with deprivation, both emotional and spiritual.

For my part, as the book winds to a close, I am aware that completing a work of love such as this is not easy because there's always the concern that something relevant is missing from the offering. Even so, I encourage you to take the knowledge you choose to extract from this book as conferring upon you the well-earned right to call yourself a *serious biocognitive student*. When challenges surface, review the applicable chapters and practice the exercises until they become a way of life. Be patient with yourself and allow others enough time to catch up with your joy. Until we meet again, I am grateful for the time and effort you invested in coauthoring excellence with an imperfect teacher. Remember, love is all you have—and all you need!

Acknowledgments

This book is a work of love and a reflection of the stellar coauthors who inspired me to write it. Some were there from the beginning, and others entered in flawless synchronicity with the drift. My son, Patrick, and my daughter, Lauren, who constantly make me proud. My mentors, John D. Bransford and George F. Solomon, who taught me how to cogently defy academic Inquisition and arrogant scientists. Loren Duffy and Sherry Hoskins, my dear friends whose love confirmed family is not limited to genetics. Jennifer Brown who brought me to Sounds True, Tami Simon who warmly welcomed me, and Sheridan McCarthy who brilliantly edited this book. Most of all, I thank Esther Barros, my mysterious woman from Uruguay who taught me how to love without fear and live my theory where it matters.

Glossary

Abundance phobia. Dysfunctional fear of success beyond the pale.

Affiliation self-esteem. The third component of self-esteem that has to do with the quality of our relationships and the people we include when we want to share our joy and good fortune. See also **valuation self-esteem** and **competence self-esteem.**

Aging. A dysfunctional assimilation of cultural portals that define how our biology "should" respond to the passing of time. See also **growing older.**

Amygdala. Two almond-shaped areas of the brain (one on each side); part of the limbic system; process memory and emotional reactions, mainly fear.

Anticipated joy. A biocognitive term to illustrate how the unknown aspect of future joy can be more anxiety-producing than known misery. See also **known misery.**

Aphaeresis. In ancient Greek, "to let go"; the tool that releases language and imagery, that gets rid of the distractions to avoid going deeper in contemplative inquiry. See also **apophasis** and **aporia.**

Apophasis. The ancient Greek word means "to say no"; saying no to the language and imagery that block transcendence into undisturbed experience, leaving you with a space void of words and imagery. See also **aphaeresis** and **aporia.**

Aporia. The ancient Greek word means "without way or passage;" the tool that helps you reach what is not possible with linguistic inquiry. See also **aphaeresis** and **apophasis.**

Archetypal wounds. The three emotional wounds inflicted by cultures: shame, abandonment, and betrayal.

Atonement archetype. A cultural or spiritual belief that one must suffer before reaching desired goals, or because of past conduct.

Belief horizons. The limits or edges of our knowing. Within the limits, information is perceived as familiar, and outside the limits it is interpreted as foreign.

Beyond the pale. Historically, early tribal cultures enclosed their members' dwellings within fences or walls ("pale") to protect against wild animals and enemies. If you remained within the enclosure, you were protected, accepted, and required to work for the collective benefit of the tribe. But if you went "beyond the pale," you were no longer considered a contributor to the benefit of the tribe, as venturing out for your own benefit did not serve tribal needs.

Biocognition. Term coined by Dr. Mario Martinez in 1998 to define his theory of mind-body-culture. In his biocognitive theory, Martinez proposes that cognition and biology coemerge within a cultural history to find maximum contextual relevance. Biocognition challenges the limitations of the conventional sciences that reduce life to its biological components and dismiss mind as a neurochemical expression. Rather than an epiphenomenon of biology, cognition coemerges with biology in an inseparable coauthorship of phenomenology and physicality within cultural horizons.

Biocognitive contemplative method. A meditation method that systematically embodies the observations by identifying where they manifest in the body as sensations and emotions.

Biocognitive immune system. More than protector, the immune system *learns* to confirm the operative consciousness you live.

Biocognitive iteration. Repeating a sequence of operations to successively expand the contextual **felt meaning** of a symbol. Each repetition of a concept adds new information to expand and deepen your felt meaning of the concept.

Bioinformation. The exchange of information by living beings, including the symbols and biological responses expressed during communication.

Bioinformational field. Mindbody information interpreted in culturally determined contexts.

Bios. Hector Sabelli found what he calls *biotic patterns* in natural processes, such as heartbeat intervals that, although chaotic in their nonlinear nature, show complex *novel patterns* rather than unpredictability. Thus, self-generating systems such as living organisms continually create novel and transient patterns that diversify in time. (See *Sabelli, H.* in the bibliography).

Biosymbol. A symbol assimilated by the biology of the recipient. Biosymbols are learned early and are mostly taught by cultural editors. For example, if you are taught that going out in the rain can make you sick, the symbol "rain" gains a stressful quality that can trigger stress hormones.

Blind-by-choice. An option to ignore or reject information based on selective perception learned in a culture. For example, choosing to smoke because it has status in a culture despite the potential damage of nicotine.

Boundaries of consciousness. The level of awareness determined by our presuppositions and beliefs. We perceive as far as the boundaries of our cultural beliefs.

Ceilings of abundance. The culturally determined limits of acceptable individual achievements in wealth, health, and love—the three components of abundance.

Coauthorship. Mutual contribution and participation with an event or a person. Communication is always a coauthored engagement; it is never a one-way process void of coupling.

Coemergence. A biocognitive term that offers a new causality in biology. Rather than the conventional assumption that life processes emerge one from another, in biocognition, causality coemerges simultaneously and is perceived sequentially.

Cognitive string. A sequence of associations imposed on our time/space to make sense of events; often imposed to unrelated events creating false cause and effect.

Competence self-esteem. The component of self-esteem that identifies how competent we are in what we do professionally and personally: how well we perform at work, at home, in relationships, and with ourselves. See **valuation self-esteem** and **affiliation self-esteem.**

Contaminated love. The entanglement of love with an archetypal wound (shame, abandonment, and betrayal) taught by a cultural editor. For example, an abusive parent inadvertently teaches that love must include abuse.

Contemplation. Observational learning without judging the observation.

Contemplative psychology. The contribution to our understanding of theology as a belief system that, rather than studying religions with a particular psychological orientation, studies the psychology within each religion. For example, instead of examining Buddhism from psychoanalytical or other theoretical perspective, it studies the psychology embedded in Buddhism.

Contextual coemergence. Attributes simultaneous cause to the biocultural histories that are exchanged between communicators (at all levels) in a shared bioinformational field that seeks maximum contextual relevance. Although the emergent upward and downward causality of academic biology may be necessary, they are not sufficient to explain the complexities of life.

Counterintuitive processes. Mindbody processes that appear to go against common sense and logical progression. For example, self-caring before caring for others increases compassion.

Covenant of safety. A foundation we establish so we may communicate the language of love without the obstruction of archetypal wounds.

Cultural editors. Authority figures that mold our identity through lessons or examples within a culture. Cultural editors influence our conception of self-worthiness and our attributes.

Cultural neuroscience. A specialty that studies how sociocultural learning influences the brain. It challenges the premise that brain function does not vary across cultures.

Cultural paradigm. A conceptual working model with inherent cultural assumptions, rules of engagement, and attributions.

Cultural portals. Culturally defined life periods of how to behave and what to expect depending on age (infancy, adolescence, adult, and old). The portals convey powerful forewarnings to maintain collective identity and tribal control with admonitions such as "You are too old for that" or "What do you expect at your age?"

Cultural psychoneuroimmunology (CPNI). A new area of research and application of PNI applying cultural anthropological principles of inquiry. CPNI takes PNI from lab research with rats to investigating human mindbody processes within their cultural contexts.

Cultural time. Comprises the attributions, rituals, admonitions, beliefs, and other horizons we interweave into the time and space of our perceptual field. While *growing older* only requires the passing of time, *aging* is significantly affected by the cultural history we embody.

Default mode. A neuroscientific term to describe a default state during decreases in neural activity. For example, when you meditate, after the mind quiets, it goes to your default mode. Biocognition teaches how to take advantage of this neuropsychological process to increase creativity and change negative operative consciousness.

Downward causality. Attributing cause from the most complex to the simplest mechanism of a living system. See also **upward causality.**

Drift. A biocognitive term to identify the synchronistic emergence of interconnectedness. The drift is nonlinear and unpredictable. It unfolds without apparent cause. Although the drift cannot be sought linearly, shifting to a discovery mode increases the probability of entering its portals.

Elevated cognitions. Honor, commitment, loyalty, dignity, modesty, admiration, honesty, fairness, and magnanimity. The cognitions required to gracefully confront your challenges.

Embodied perception. The sensations, emotions, and cognition experienced when perceiving. The mindbody coauthoring that takes place during perception.

Embodied release. To let go of a belief or symbol with all its felt meaning. An experiential release of the emotions, sensations, and thoughts affected by the condition.

Embody. To identify how and where cognition is experienced in the body and the role the body plays in shaping the mind within a cultural context.

Empathic joy. An expansive concept of joy. Empathic joy teaches you to relish the achievements of others as your own, and allows you to celebrate your good fortune without fear of banishment from the tribe.

Empowerment. The capacity to access resources to overcome a challenge without compromising wellness of self and others.

Exalted emotions. Compassion, empathy, kindness, generosity, and gratitude. The emotions required to lovingly confront your challenges.

Feedforward. An out-of-order event in the present with unfolding meaning or relevance in the future. A component of interconnectedness.

Felt meaning. The mindbody experience elicited by words, images, and symbols. What you feel physically and emotionally.

Field. In biocognitive theory, an expression of the mindbody that cannot be separated from its cultural interpretation.

Field horizon. The permeable external parameters of a bioinformational field.

Fight-or-flight response. Physiological response to confront or run from a predator.

Five portals of health. Five areas of the mindbody space that manifest our most essential biosymbols, ranging from our need for safety to our quest for spirituality; gates of expression of the total being rather than reducible physical locations. They are safety, love, expression, peace, and spirit.

fMRI. Scanning (functional magnetic resonance imaging) device that shows brain activity in real time, like looking at a video of a brain to see how it responds to specified conditions.

Forgiveness. The mindbody forgiveness process has two sequential stages: the first reinstates your empowerment and the second your worthiness. When you recall and embody the felt meaning of the healing field corresponding to your wound, you experience the *alpha event:* recognition of your goodness so you may recover your sense of empowerment that has been depleted by the misdeed. Whereas in the alpha event you recognize your deeds of honor, commitment, and loyalty, in the *omega event* you feel grateful for recognizing them. Recognition of your goodness reinstates your empowerment, and gratitude recovers your worthiness. The alpha event begins your liberation and the omega event completes it.

Fusiform gyrus. An area of the brain (temporal lobe) that has to do with recognizing familiar faces; it also recognizes things we love and do well. It identifies a range of functions we cannot detect when we study the damaged brain.

Growing older. A natural process of time passing that we all experience. Although there are some physiological changes, they do not necessarily have to be pathological. See also **aging.**

Guardian of the heart. Reciprocal emotional guardianship in relationships that celebrates the union of two individuals who commit to a **covenant of**

safety to promote mutual emotional healing and resolve the fear of being wounded again. An indirect way to learn worthiness, commitment, and faith, all through the power of coauthoring love.

Healing fields. Honor, commitment, and loyalty; the antidotes to archetypal wounds of shame, abandonment, and betrayal, respectively.

Helplessness. Consistent inaccessibility to resources needed to overcome a challenge.

Horizons. The fluid parameters that delineate a bioinformational field. Unlike rigid boundaries, horizons are permeable and allow information exchange between bioinformational fields.

Horizontal lover. A horizontal lover seeks quantity, is emotionally shallow, and views their most recent "soul mate" as a temporary experience of intensity, to be traded in for another one when the partner begins to demand emotional substance. Horizontal lovers are committed to noncommitment. They have many acquaintances and few friends. Their archetypal wounds run deep, and when they surface, these lovers usually project them onto others rather than take ownership. See also **vertical lover.**

HPA axis. See **stress axis.**

IgA (Immunoglobulin type A). An antibody secreted by B cells that fights upper respiratory infections such as the common cold. The IgAs can be triggered by observing and expressing acts of kindness and compassion.

Imperfection wisdom. Extracted wisdom from approximations to perfection. In the process of reaching a goal, mistakes are viewed as portals to valuable information.

Imperfection paradox. Choosing unwanted imperfection to avoid the perfection you yearn for, but lack the self-worth to accept.

Implicate consciousness. The collective knowledge that surfaces into awareness based on the demands of cultural contexts.

Incidental learning. The process of learning something wherein you coincidentally learn competence in something else.

Indeterminate locality. A biocognitive term to conceptualize how nonlinear communication is archived through multiple complexity localities that are not accessible until they **coemerge** into linear processes. Indeterminate locality provides an alternative to the improper use of quantum nonlocality when defining nonlinearity. Quantum nonlocality has no **travel origin** and it applies to subatomic particles, whereas indeterminate locality has complex multiplicity of travel origins and takes place above atomic levels. While indeterminate locality is based on complexity theory, nonlocality is a quantum physics event. It is an error of category to use these two terms interchangeably.

Intellectual forgiveness. A helpless imposition of mind over emotion. Relying on reasoning and excluding the experiential components of the misdeed you want to forgive.

Intimate language of love. The expression of love based on how it is taught by cultural editors.

Investment value. The implicit worth given to an intention, event, or action.

Joy fingerprint. The unique things that excite you individually and make you come alive.

Known misery. Negative habits and lifestyles that become a way of life without attempting to change conditions. See also **anticipated joy.**

Languages of inquiry. The three languages of inquiry, each of which has a range of function: *descriptive, prescriptive,* and *evocative.* Their names illustrate what they do. For example, knowing an apple: the descriptive language teaches you apples are red and round; prescriptive explains you can eat them raw or cooked; evocative must be experienced because it awakens (evokes) a particular state of reality in which description and prescription will not suffice. When you hold and taste an apple, it *evokes* flavor, aroma, roundness, and weightiness. In biocognition terms, the evocative language illustrates the experience of coauthoring within a bioinformational field.

Laudable field. A bioinformational field of **elevated cognitions** and **exalted emotions.**

Ledger relationship. A relationship where partners focus on keeping score, giving while expecting to receive and taking while expecting to give back. Although this type of exchange may seem reasonable, when you look deeper, you see transactions of giving and taking with hidden agendas rather than offering and receiving for the pure joy of experiencing the exchange.

Limpu. Name given by Bolivian shamans to the symptoms of asthma when a person has witnessed a stillbirth. The shamanic diagnosis declares the "illness" is incurable because the spirit of the stillborn, in order to remain on earth, must inhabit the patient's body and consume it.

Lived theory. Living a theory entails embodying its principles in the form of actions. To sustain a change to live the theory, actions must become rituals.

Mature tolerance. To honor the conduct of others without shaming our own.

Meaningful nothingness. Since words can only be defined by other words, you can't explain deeper levels of consciousness without creating contradictions; when you also remove images, you end up with what contemplatives call meaningful nothingness.

Meeting of horizons. The intercommunication between two bioinformational fields. The horizons are the permeable boundaries of fields that assimilate or reject new bioinformation.

Middle way. A Buddhist psychological concept meaning optimal position between opposites.

Mindbody. The inseparable coemergence of mind and body. A **coauthoring** of thoughts and biology shaped by their cultural history.

Mindful rituals. Periodic behaviors without excess or harmful effects that identify us with our culture and our joy. For example, having tea in the morning while reflecting on the day to come; a daily walk; or taking a nap. See also **mindless needs.**

Mindless needs. Habitual and excessive behavior based on external needs. We only abuse what we mindlessly need and not what we mindfully love. See also **mindful rituals.**

Novelty kindness. Drawing from love to find novelty in boring reruns; a key to shifting from **novelty plateaus** and letting creativity fly.

Novelty plateau. Repetitive patterns in yourself and your partner that can dampen your enthusiasm. Just as markets have periods of contraction after consistent growth, our journey of **vertical love** has novelty plateaus at which we tire of communication that has lost its initial function. What was initially witty has lost its funny punch line, what was once refreshing has turned stale, and what was exciting has become predictable.

Novelty. Whatever emerges for the first time is novel; the new; in complexity theory, novelty is a unique condition of recurrence between chaos and randomness that can be measured by quantifying the scarcity of recurrences.

Oxytocin. A hormone and neurotransmitter produced mainly in the pituitary gland. It has gained popularity because of its association with bonding, monogamy, and love. This does not mean, however, that those behaviors are *caused by* oxytocin.

Paradigm. A conceptual working model with inherent assumptions, rules of engagement, and attributions.

Perceptual investment value. The implicit worth given to an intention, event, or action.

Portals. Gates of expression of the total being rather than reducible physical locations. For example, the brain is a portal rather than the physical locality of thoughts. Portals are expressions of the bioinformational field.

Prayer of quiet. A contemplative method and not a prayer, associated with St. Teresa of Avila, a sixteenth-century Catholic nun. She warned that God cannot be known with our faculties (cognition) because we are not prepared to handle the intensity of the experience. The prayer of quiet teaches you to drop your ego and create a place of quiet where God can bestow his wisdom. But the objective is to invite God to the place of quiet, not to seek him.

Primitive emotions. Emotions founded in dysfunctional fear that are on the side opposite to the **exalted emotions**. Fear is a physiological response that is necessary to signal danger and warn us to proceed with caution, but other than those adaptive functions, it does not serve us well because it alienates us from love. If we embrace it beyond its adaptive purpose, it grows into anger, hatred, jealousy, resentment, envy, greed, shame, and other primitive emotions that disconnect us from the best we have to offer.

Pristine love. Love, free of entangled archetypal wounds. The offering and receiving of love without attachments of shame, abandonment, or betrayal.

Prolepsis. An enigmatic term from the Greek, defined as a preconception; the anachronistic representation of something existing before its proper or historical time.

Psychoneuroimmunology. An interdisciplinary field that investigates the connection between behavior and the immune, nervous, and endocrine systems.

Recontextualize. To change the felt meaning of a belief, emotion, and context.

Relational incompleteness. In order to learn, you have to *relate* what you want to know. You have to relate maleness with femaleness to know your gender, tallness with shortness to know your height. But most concepts you want to know cannot be known completely.

Ritual. A behavior or event that gives inclusive meaning to the individual, family, or culture. For example, breaking bread with family, celebrating birthdays and holidays with family. A ritual identifies what we are about and our belongingness in a culture.

Routine. A behavior or event that reflects what one must do with some regularity. For example, going to work, taking a shower, or grocery shopping. A routine identifies what we must do to maintain the status quo.

Segments of nothingness. The experience in between thoughts and observations during contemplative practices; segments without contexts.

Self-referent fallacy. The interpretation of the actions or circumstances of others based on our own experiences.

Self-worthiness. The value you assign to your identity based on your personal accomplishments and feedback from your cultural editors.

Serial commitment. Commitment to a partner instead of commitment to longevity with a partner.

Shifts and gaps. A biocognitive contemplative technique that teaches how to shift back and forth from a negative to a positive condition. According to biocognitive theory, mindbody recontextualizing takes place in the gap between shifts.

Stress axis. When we experience a stressful condition, although the process is complex and is not limited to the brain, the hypothalamus secretes corticotropic releasing hormones (CRH) to the pituitary, which then releases adrenocorticotropic hormone (ACTH) to the adrenal glands, which in turn release cortisol (C). This chain of hormonal secretion is called the HPA axis, to describe the three types of glands involved; the hypothalamus and the pituitary are single glands in the brain, and the adrenals are a pair, located on top of the kidneys.

Synchronicity. Meaningful coincidental and out-of-order events. The meaningful coincidences are always there to unfold when you follow the **drift** and enter a portal of synchronicity. But since the portals are tentative and hidden from linear order, you can't seek them directly or at will. You must wait for an invitation to detour using a different navigational compass.

Travel origin. Identifiable beginning place of a trajectory.

Tumor necrosis factor (TNF). Molecule that is a reliable indicator of inflammation, usually triggered by infection and other immunological damage. PNI research shows TNF can be triggered by the emotion of shame.

Unselfing. A biocognitive term to express the process of detaching from the social and cultural labels of self. Unselfing occurs during deep levels of meditation or contemplative states. It is a groundless awareness that rids self of all its masks and labels. Without proper guidance, unselfing can be a frightening experience. In pathological processes, it manifests as dissociative and depersonalization states during extreme anxiety reactions. Contemplative adepts can enter unselfing states at will.

Undulation. The ripple after-effects of a nonphysical process; awareness without context.

Upward causality. Attributing cause from the simplest to the most complex mechanism of a living system. See also **downward causality.**

Valuation self-esteem. How much joy we can experience from our positive deeds and fortuitous circumstances. But we must feel valuable before we can appreciate the value of a circumstance. See also **competence self-esteem** and **affiliation self-esteem.**

Vertical lover. Vertical lovers seek quality and emotional depth; they take soul mates for better or for worse until death. This does not mean they remain in abusive or toxic relationships—this is *co*authorship, not a one-way street. Vertical lovers never cease to find novelty in their partners.

Witnessing. Observing without interpreting. Allowing information to surface from consciousness without categorizing it.

Bibliography

Ader, Robert, ed. *Psychoneuroimmunology.* 4th ed. San Diego: Academic Press, 2006.

Austin, J. H. *Zen-Brain Reflections: Reviewing Recent Developments in Meditation and States of Consciousness.* Cambridge: MIT Press, 2006.

Bach-y-Rita, P. *Brain Mechanisms in Sensory Substitution.* New York: Academic Press, 1972.

Bohn, D. *Wholeness and the Implicate Order.* London: Ark, 1983.

Bourdieu, P. *La Creencia y el Cuerpo, en El Sentido Práctico.* Madrid: Taurus, 1980.

Brody, H. *The Placebo Response: How You Can Release the Body's Inner Pharmacy for Better Health.* New York: Cliff Street Books, 2000.

Chiao, J. Y., ed. *Cultural Neuroscience: Cultural Influences on Brain Function.* New York: Elsevier, 2009.

Citro, S. "La Antropología del Cuerpo y los Cuerpos en-el-mundo. Inicios para Una Genealogía Indisciplinar." In *Cuerpos Plurales: Antropología de y desde los Cuerpos,* edited by Silvia Citro, 17–58. Buenos Aires: Biblos, 2011.

Clayton, K. and B. Frey. "Fractal memory for visual form." Paper presented at the annual convention of the Society for Chaos Theory in Psychology and Life Sciences, Berkeley, California, June 1996.Cohen, Irun R. *Tending Adam's Garden: Evolving the Cognitive Immune Self.* New York: Academic Press, 2000.

Colombetti, G. *The Feeling Body: Affective Science Meets the Enactive Mind.* Cambridge: MIT Press, 2013.

Combs, A. *The Radiance of Being: Complexity, Chaos and the Evolution of Consciousness.* St. Paul: Paragon House, 1996.

Crandon-Malamud, L. "Phantoms and Physicians: Social Change Through Medical Pluralism." In *The Anthropology of Medicine,* edited by L. Romanucci-Ross, et al. London: Bergin & Garvey, 1997, 31–53.

————. *From the Fat of our Souls: Social Change, Political Process, and Medical Pluralism in Bolivia.* Berkeley: University of California Press, 1991.

Csordas, T. "Embodiment, Agency, Sexual Difference, and Illness." In *A Companion to the Anthropology of the Body and Embodiment,* edited by Frances Mascia-Lees. Chichester, UK: John Wiley and Sons, 2011, 137–56.

————. "The Body's Career in Anthropology." In *Anthropological Theory Today,* edited by Henrietta Moore. Cambridge, UK: Holilty Press, 1999, 172–205.

————. *Embodiment and Experience: The Existential Ground of Culture and Self.* Cambridge: Cambridge University Press, 1995.

————. "Embodiment as a Paradigm for Anthropology." *Ethos,* Vol. 18, no. 1 (1990): 5–47.

Dalai Lama. *Transforming the Mind.* London: Thorsons, 2000.

Daruna, J. H. *Introduction to Psychoneuroimmunology.* San Diego: Elsevier, 2004.

Davidson, R. *The Emotional Life of Your Brain: How Its Unique Patterns Affect the Way You Think, Feel, and Live—and How You Can Change Them.* New York: Penguin, 2012.

de Wit, H. F. *The Spiritual Path: An Introduction to the Psychology of Spiritual Traditions.* Pittsburgh: Duquesne University Press, 1994.

————. *Contemplative Psychology.* Pittsburgh: Duquesne University Press, 1991.

Dickerson, S., M. E. Kemeny, N. Aziz, K. Kim, and J. L. Fahey. "Immunological Effects of Induced Shame and Guilt." *Psychosomatic Medicine* 66 (2004): 124–31.

Dickerson, S., and M. E. Kemeny. "Acute Stressors and Cortisol Responses: A Theoretical Integration and Synthesis of Laboratory Research." *Psychological Bulletin* 130, no. 3 (2004): 355–91.

Dossey, L. *Healing Words: The Power of Prayer and the Practice of Medicine.* New York: HarperCollins, 1993.

Eckhart, M. *The Essential Sermons, Commentaries, Treatises and Defense.* Mahwah, NJ: Paulist Press, 1981.

Finnegan, J. *The Audacity of Spirit: The Meaning and Shaping of Spirituality Today.* Dublin: Veritas Publications, 2008.

Hahn, R. A. *Sickness and Healing: An Anthropological Perspective.* New Haven, CT: Yale University Press, 1995.

Hahn, R. A. and A. M. Kleinman. "Belief as Pathogen, Belief as Medicine: 'Voodoo Death' and the Placebo Phenomenon in Anthropological Perspective." *Medical Anthropology Quarterly,* Vol. 14, no. 3 (1983): 16–19.

Hay, D. *Something There: The Biology of the Human Spirit.* Philadelphia: Templeton Foundation Press, 2007.

Heidegger, M. *On Time and Being.* Chicago: University of Chicago Press, 1972.

Held, R. "Shifts in Binaural Localization after Prolonged Exposures to Atypical Combinations of Stimuli." *American Journal of Psychology,* Vol. 68 (1955): 526–48.

Held, R. and A. Hein. "Adaptation of Disarranged Hand-Eye Coordination Contingent upon Re-Afferent Stimulation." *Perceptual and Motor Skills* Vol. 8 (1958): 87–90.

Hoffman, M. L. *Empathy and Moral Development: Implications for Caring and Justice.* Cambridge: Cambridge University Press, 2000.

Jenkins, J. "Bodily Transactions of the Passions: El Calór among Salvadoran Women Refugees." In *Embodiment and Experience,* edited by Thomas J. Csordas. Cambridge: Cambridge University Press, 1994, 163–182.

Kapur, N., ed. *The Paradoxical Brain.* Cambridge: Cambridge University Press, 2011.

Keysers, C. *The Empathic Brain.* Social Brain Press, 2011.

Kierkegaard, S. *The Concept of Anxiety.* Princeton: Princeton University Press, 1980.

————. *The Sickness unto Death.* Princeton: Princeton University Press, 1980.

Koenig, H. G. and J. C. Harvey. *The Link between Religion and Health: Psychoneuroimmunology and the Faith Factor.* Oxford: Oxford University Press, 2002.

Langer, E. *Counterclockwise: Mindful Health and the Power of Possibility.* New York: Ballantine Books, 2009.

Laughlin. C. D. *Brain, Symbol & Experience: Toward a Neurophenomenology of Human Consciousness.* Berkeley: Shambhala, 1990.

Levent, N. and A. Pascual-Leone. *The Multisensory Museum: Cross-Disciplinary Perspectives on Touch, Sound, Smell, Memory, and Space.* New York: Rowman & Littlefield, 2014.

Lieberman, M. D., et al. "Putting Feelings into Words: Affect Labeling Disrupts Amygdala Activity to Affective Stimuli." *Psychological Science,* Vol. 18, no. 5 (2007): 421–28.

Lock, M. *An Anthropology of Biomedicine.* New York: Wiley-Blackwell, 2010.

Low, S. M. "Embodied Metaphors: Nerves as Lived Experience." In *Embodiment and Experience,* edited by Thomas J. Csordas, 139–82. Cambridge: Cambridge University Press, 1994.

Malafouris, L. *How Things Shape the Mind: A Theory of Material Engagement.* Cambridge: MIT Press, 2013.

Martinez, M. E. "Hacia un Nuevo Modelo del Sistema Inmunológico: El Gran Confirmador de la Conciencia Corporizada que Vivimos." In *Bases de la Inmunología Clínica,* edited by J. L. Aguilar, 700–18. Lima, Perú: Ed. Hamex & AM, 2013.

————. "Hacia un Nuevo Modelo del Sistema Inmune: El Gran Confirmador." In *El Padecimiento Mental: Entre la Salud y la Enfermedad,* edited by A. Trimboli, J. C. Fantin, et al., 139–42. Buenos Aires: AASM, 2009.

————. *The MindBody Code: How the Mind Wounds and Heals the Body.* CD. Louisville, CO: Sounds True, 2009.

————. "The Biocognition of Personal Ethics: Does the Immune System Have Morals?" Paper presented at the Ninth International Conference on Ethics across the Curriculum, Milltown Institute, Dublin, Ireland, November 2007.

————. "A Biocultural Model of Aging." *Kybernetes,* Vol. 32, no. 5/6 (2003): 653–57.

————. "Effectiveness of Operationalized Gestalt Therapy Role-Playing in the Treatment of Phobic Behaviors." *Gestalt Review,* Vol. 6, no. 2 (2002): 148–67.

————. "The Process of Knowing: A Biocognitive Epistemology." *The Journal of Mind and Behavior,* Vol. 22, no. 4, (2001): 407–26.

Maturana, H., and F. Varela. *Autopoiesis and Cognition.* Boston: D. Reidel, 1980.

May, G. G. *The Dark Night of the Soul.* New York: HarperCollins, 2005.

McClelland, D. C. "Motivational Factors in Health and Disease." *American Psychologist,* Vol. 44 (1989): 675–83.

McClelland, D. C. and C. Kirshnit. "The Effect of Motivational Arousal through Films on Salivary Immunoglobulin A." *Psychology and Health* 2, (1988): 31–52.

McGonigal, K. *The Willpower Instinct.* New York: Avery Trade, 2013.

Merleau-Ponty, M. *Phenomenology of Perception.* London: Routledge and Kegan Ltd, 1962.

Moerman, D. E. "General Medical Effectiveness and Human Biology: Placebo Effects in the Treatment of Ulcer Disease." *Medical Anthropological Quarterly,* Vol. 14, no. 3 (1983): 13–16.

Nietzsche, F. *Beyond Good and Evil: Prelude to a Philosophy of the Future.* New York: Dover Publications, 1997.

Pennebaker, J., ed. *Emotion, Disclosure and Health.* Washington, DC: American Psychological Association, 2007.

Phillips, D. P., et al. "The Hound of the Baskervilles Effect: Natural Experiment on the Influence of Psychological Stress on the Timing of Death." *British Journal of Medicine,* Vol. 323 (2001): 1443–446.

Ponticus, E. *Ad Monachos.* New York: The Newman Press, 2003.

Ricouer, P. *From Text to Action: Essays on Hermeneutics, II.* Evanston, IL: Northwestern University Press, 2007.

Sabelli, H. "Trigonometric Chaos and Bios." Paper presented at the Eleventh Annual International Conference of the Society for Chaos Theory in Psychology and Life Sciences, Madison, Wisconsin, August 2001.

Sacks, O. *The Man Who Mistook His Wife for a Hat.* New York: Touchstone, 1998.

Segall, M. H., et al. *The Influence of Culture on Visual Perception.* Bobbs-Merrill, 1966.

Solomon, G. F. *From Psyche to Soma and Back: Tales of Biopsychosocial Medicine.* Philadelphia: Xlibris Corp, 2000.

Solomon, G. F. and R. H. Moos. "The Relationship of Personality to the Presence of Rheumatoid Factor in Asymptomatic Relatives of Patients with Rheumatoid Arthritis." *Psychosomatic Medicine,* Vol. 27 (1965): 350–60.

Ramachandran, V. S. *The Tell-Tale Brain.* New York: W. W. Norton, 2012.

St. Teresa of Avila. *Interior Castle.* New York: Image Books, 1989.

Tauber, A. I. *The Immune Self: Theory or Metaphor?* Cambridge: Cambridge University Press, 1994.

Varela, F. *El Fenómeno de la Vida*. Santiago, Chile: Comunicaciones Noreste Ltda, 2000.

Varela, F., E. Thompson, and E. Rorsch. *The Embodied Mind: Cognitive Science and Human Experience*. Cambridge: MIT Press, 1991.

Wallace, B. A. *Contemplative Science*. New York: Columbia University Press, 2007.

Walsh, V., A. Pascual-Leone, and S. M. Kosslyn. *Transcranial Magnetic Stimulation: A Neurochronometrics of Mind*. Bradford, 2005.

Ware, N. "Toward a Model of Social Course in Chronic Illness: The Example of Chronic Fatigue Syndrome." *Culture, Medicine, and Psychiatry,* Vol. 23 (1999): 303–31.

Wilce, J. M. *Social and Cultural Lives of Immune Systems*. London: Routledge, 2003.

Wilson, C. *The Outsider*. New York: Tarcher-Putnam, 1982.

Index

by cultural editors, 153–54, 155
cultural history and, 151–55
disempowerment and, 150–51
forgiveness and, 150
interpretation of, 151
loss of innocence and, 155–56
perpetrator of, biocognitive space of,
    152–55, 156

Zen koans, 180

About the Author

Mario E. Martinez, PsyD, is a US clinical neuropsychologist who lectures worldwide on how cultural beliefs affect health and longevity. In his theory of biocognitive science, he offers a new paradigm that investigates the causes of health and the learning of illnesses. Biocognition identifies complex discoveries of how our cultural beliefs affect our immune, nervous, and endocrine systems, and translates them to practical applications. He is the proponent of cultural psychoneuroimmunology and has published numerous articles on the causes of health based on his research with centenarians from five different continents. Dr. Martinez has investigated cases of alleged stigmata for the Catholic Church, the BBC, National Geographic, and the Discovery Channel. He loves to cook, travel, and windsurf. He lives in Montevideo, Uruguay.

About Sounds True

S ounds True is a multimedia publisher whose mission is to inspire and support personal transformation and spiritual awakening. Founded in 1985 and located in Boulder, Colorado, we work with many of the leading spiritual teachers, thinkers, healers, and visionary artists of our time. We strive with every title to preserve the essential "living wisdom" of the author or artist. It is our goal to create products that not only provide information to a reader or listener, but that also embody the quality of a wisdom transmission.

For those seeking genuine transformation, Sounds True is your trusted partner. At SoundsTrue.com you will find a wealth of free resources to support your journey, including exclusive weekly audio interviews, free downloads, interactive learning tools, and other special savings on all our titles.

To learn more, please visit SoundsTrue.com/freegifts or call us toll free at 800-333-9185.

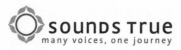